THE SIRTFOOD DIET:

A Beginner's Guide To Weight Loss.
Activate Your Skinny Gene, Boost
Metabolism, And Burn Fat. Including Tips
To Prepare A Sirtfood Meal Plan.

© Copyright 2020 - All rights reserved.

Table Of Contents

Introduction

U nlike fasting, the Sirtfood diet doesn't involve skipping meals in order to experience the benefits it can offer. Therefore, you are not going through starvation to reach your weight loss and health goals. The diet involves calorie restriction meaning, you lower the number of calories you consume on a daily basis, but you will still have breakfast, lunch, dinner, and even desserts or snacks. Now you are probably wondering, "How am I going to lose pounds by eating three meals a day?" The secret lies within the meal plan, as it can seriously deliver amazing results.

The founders of the diet promise that you will lose seven pounds in the first seven days. This may sound too good to be true, but it is clinically proven. Not all bodies react the same to this diet so that the weight loss can be more or less visible. This diet promises to deliver, so you will have outstanding results for trying it. Since you will feel a lot more energized compared to your normal diet, why not put the excess energy to good use? Plenty of athletes from the UK have tried this diet, so you can easily conclude that it works perfectly fine with training and workout. In order to maximize the fat-burning effect, I would highly recommend workouts, but it is up to you how intense you want to train.

When you are satisfied with the weight you lost so far, you can simply go into the maintenance phase of this diet. Sounds neat, right? This is what's great about this diet — it gives you the possibility to preserve your weight, unlike many other radical diets. Most people following a diet complain that they start to gain weight immediately after quitting the diet. These radical diets don't have a preservation mode, so they don't give you the chance to enjoy the weight you lost.

This diet has some major advantages compared to other meal plans or programs designed to lose weight and get healthier.

The ingredients are very familiar, and you can easily combine them with other foods that are not rich in sirtuins.

Also, this diet is very permissive. You can try plenty of food out there, and you are not too limited to veggies and fruits. If you are used to eating a lot, then you might think of compensating when eating these foods just to get you satisfied. There might be people trying sirtfoods and not losing weight. In this case, their problem lies within the form, variety, and quantity. It is very hard to have a meal consisting only of sirtfoods I'm referring to main meals, not snacks or desserts, so you need to find the right balance between sirtfoods and normal food. Having regular meals is very important because if you don't have the meals within a set timeframe, the diet might not work. The general rule about not eating too much at dinner or having dinner late in the evening applies.

Let's try to understand the secret of these sirtfoods. What exactly do they contain that activates sirtuins? Arugula contains nutrients like kaempferol and quercetin, capable of activating sirtuins. Buckwheat contains rutting. Capers have the same nutrients as arugula. Celery has luteolin and apigenin. Cocoa contains epicatechin. Chilies have a higher concentration of myricetin and luteolin. Coffee contains caffeic acid. Widely used in the Mediterranean diet, the extra-virgin olive oil has hydroxytyrosol and oleuropein. Kale contains the same nutrients as arugula and capers. You can find ajoene and myricetin in garlic. In green tea, you can find EGCG epigallocatechin gallate. Medjool dates contain caffeic and Gallic acid. Parsley has myricetin and apigenin. In red endives, you can find luteolin. Quercetin can be found in red onions. Strawberries contain fisetin. Walnuts are a great source of Gallic acid. Turmeric has cur cumin. Soy contains formononetin and daidzein. Red wine has piceatannol and resveratrol.

Now you are probably wondering why I'm bothering you with these fancy names of nutrients. Indeed, they all have the power to trigger sirtuins, but as it turns out, our standard diet is very poor when it comes to these nutrients. Researchers have proven that a standard US diet only contains 13 milligrams daily value of five key sirtuin-activating nutrients apigenin, luteolin, kaempferol, myricetin, and quercetin. In Japan, daily intake is five times higher. Well, a proper Sirtfood diet should allow you to consume hundreds of milligrams of these important ingredients per day. Obviously, if you manage to introduce most of the ingredients and sirtfoods mentioned above into your daily meal plan, you can effectively reap the benefits of this diet.

The nutrients mentioned above should be consumed in a natural state. This is how this diet works. You may not have the same effects if you take supplements, as the body absorbs and assimilates them a lot better in their natural form. If you take, for instance, resveratrol, this nutrient is poorly absorbed in a supplement form. However, if you consume it in a natural form, the absorption is six times higher. This should now encourage you to drink a lot of red wine. A glass of it should be more than enough. But when it comes to drinks, you need to have coffee and green tea on a daily basis. You don't have to replace water with green tea, but it is very good to have green tea a few times per day.

It is good to have as many of these sirtfoods as possible to make sure you are getting the necessary intake of sirtuin-activating nutrients. Most of them are very common or familiar, and this is the beauty of the Sirtfood diet. Therefore, it is not something extraordinary to eat garlic or red onion, strawberries, blueberries, or walnuts. It is highly recommended to make sure you include turmeric in your diet, as well.

When it comes to consuming fruits and veggies, most nutritionists would agree that it is best to consume them fresh and raw. Eat them directly. This is how you will get all the nutrients and vitamins from them, and you will not lose anything. However, when it comes to leafy greens, it is better to juice them, as this procedure removes the low-nutrient fiber from them and allows you to have a super concentrated dose of sirtuin-activating polyphenols.

We have talked about the form and variety of the sirtfoods. Another important fact when it comes to this diet is the schedule of your meals. The Sirtfood diet should fit exactly in your busy schedule, but you need to remember to eat as early as possible in the morning.

Since this diet allows you to eat plenty of foods, it rocks when it comes to diversity. This is why you can simply feel free to consume meat, fish, and seafood if you want. As a general rule of thumb, consume less red meat beef and pork and more poultry, fish, and seafood.

The Sirtfood diet should slowly become your default meal plan. Therefore, you don't have to stick just to the four-week meal plan. Sirtuins need to be in your diet every day of the week, so why stop after finishing the fourth week? If you have a good thing running, you really don't need to interrupt it. Plus, the longer you are following this diet, the more health benefits you will experience. Sounds great, right? This should be the ultimate motivation to make you try the Sirtfood diet on a regular basis. You need to check yourself whether or not you want to prevent or even reverse some of the most common diseases caused by poor diet, slow down your aging process, and lose some weight while doing it. If it's a yes, then you need to try this diet now!

CHAPTER 1:

Sirtfood Diet Theory

The Sirtfood diet attempts to emulate the advantages of fasting diets, but without any of the drawbacks. Here, you will learn about the theory of fasting diets and how the Sirtfood diet cleverly achieves the same effect, but without any of the actual fasting.

Many fasting diets have become popular in the past five years. The most well-known are the several variants of the intermittent fasting structure, such as the five-two diet. In the five-two diet, you fast during the weekend and eat normally during the working days of the week. These diets have proven and demonstrated effects on longevity, weight loss and overall health.

This is because these fasting diets activate the 'skinny gene' in our body. This gene causes the fat storage processes to shut down and for the body to enter a state of 'survival' mode, which in turn causes the body to burn fat.

Burning fat is what you might expect if you essentially start starving yourself, but another interesting effect of fasting is that your body switches from the replication of cells to the repair of cells.

Anytime cells in your body replicate there is a small chance of your DNA being damaged in the process. However if your body repairs dying and older cells there is no risk of DNA damage, which is the reason why fasting is associated with lower prevalence of degenerative disease, such as Alzheimer's.

However, the problem with fasting diets, as the name implies, is that you have to fast. Fasting feels awful, especially when we are surrounded by other people having regular eating habits. It also puts some social spotlight on your own diet – explaining to your co-workers or your extended family why you are not eating on certain days is bound to generate incredulity and challenges to your diet regime.

Furthermore, even though fasting has numerous associated benefits, there are some downsides too. Fasting is associated with muscle loss, as the body doesn't discriminate between muscle mass and fat tissue when choosing cells to burn for energy.

Fasting also risks malnutrition, simply by not eating enough foods to get essential nutrients. This risk can be somewhat alleviated by taking vitamin supplements and eating nutrient rich foods, but fasting can also slow and halt the digestive system altogether – preventing the absorption of supplements. These supplements also need dietary fat to be dissolved, which you might also lack if you were to implement a strict fasting method.

On top of this, fasting isn't appropriate for a huge range of people. Obviously, you don't want children to fast and potentially inhibit their growth. Likewise, the elderly, the ill and the pregnant are all just too vulnerable to the risks of fasting.

Additionally, there are several psychological detriments to fasting, despite commonly being associated with spiritual revelations. Fasting makes you irritable and causes you to feel slightly on edge – your body is telling you constantly that you need to forage for food, enacting physical processes that affect your mood and emotions.

This is why the authors of the Sirtfood diet sought a replacement for fasting diets. Fasting is clearly beneficial for our body, but it just isn't practical for society at large. This is where sirtuin activators and Sirtfoods come to the rescue.

Sirtuins were first discovered in 1984 in yeast molecules. Of course, once it became apparent that sirtuin activators affected a variety of factors, such as lifespan and metabolic activity, interest in these proteins blossomed.

Sirtuin activators boost your mitochondria's activity, the part of the biological cell which is responsible for the production of energy. This in turn mirrors the energy-boosting effects which also occur due to exercise and fasting. The sirtfood diet is thought to start a process called adipogenesis, which prevents fat cells from duplicating – which should interest any potential dieter.

The interesting part is that the sirtuin activators actually influence your genetics. The notion of the 'genetic' lottery is embedded in the public consciousness, but genes are actually more changeable then you might think. You won't be able to change your eye color, or your height, but you can activate or de-activate certain genes based on environmental factors. This is called epigenetics and it is a fascinating field of study.

Sirtuin activators cause the SIR genes to activate, the before-mentioned 'skinny genes', which in turn increases the release of sirts. Sirts, or Silent Information Regulators also help regulate the circadian rhythm, which is your natural body clock and influences sleep patterns.

Sleep is important for many vital biological processes, including those that help regulate blood sugar (which is also important for losing weight). If you find yourself constantly stuck in a state of lag and brain fog, this may be caused by your circadian rhythm being out of sync, which is another way the sirtfood diet can help your body.

Additionally, sirts help contain free radicals. Free radicals are not as awesome as the sound – they are A.W.O.L particles in your body that damage your DNA and speed up the ageing process.

To summarize, the Sirtfood diet contains foods which are high in sirtuin activators. Sirtuin activators activate your SIR genes, or 'skinny genes' which enact beneficial metabolic processes.

These processes, which involve molecules, called Sirts, causes your body to burn fat, repair bodily cells and combat free radicals.

Evidence

So, sirtfoods have been hailed as another dietary wonder – but where is the cold, hard evidence? Well, the evidence for the sirtfood diet comes from multiple sources. To start with, Aidan Goggins and Glen Matten, the originators of the Sirtfood diet, performed their own trial at a privately owned fitness center to test sirtfoods themselves.

At a fitness center called KX, in Chelsea, London the two authors of the sirtfood diet made a selection of their clientele eat a carefully monitored constructed sirtfood diet. What is generally fascinating about the study is that weight wasn't the only variable measured – the researchers also measured body composition and metabolic activity – they were searching for the holistic effect of the diet.

97.5% of people managed to stick to the first-three day fasting period, involving only 1000 calories. Generally speaking, this is a much higher rate of success than typical fasting diets, where many people have their willpower shattered in just the first few days.

Out of the 40 participants, 39 completed the study. In terms of overall fitness and weight, the individuals in the study were well distributed – 2 were officially obese, 15 fell into the overweight category whilst 22 had a regular body mass index. There were also 21 women and 18 men – a diet for both the genders! However, with that being said, being members of a fitness center the individuals in the study were more likely to exercise more than the standard population – a potential confounding factor.

Participants lost over 7lbs on average in the first week. Every participant experienced an improvement in body composition, even if their gains were not as dramatic as their peers.

There were also numerous reported psychological benefits, although these were not formally quantified.

These improvements include an overall sense of feeling and looking better. As a side note, it was also claimed the 40 participants rarely felt hungry, even despite the calorie deficits imposed by the diet.

The most startling result from the sirtfood diet is that muscle mass after the 1-week diet period was either the same as before, or showed slight improvements. Dieting law typically states that when losing fat, muscle is also lost, usually around 20-30% of the total weight loss, you should lose 2-3 lbs. of muscle for every 10 lbs. lost.

Of course, retaining muscle isn't just better from an overall fitness perspective, but also from an aesthetic view. A common fear, especially in men, is that if they lose weight is that they will look skinny, scrawny and unhealthy. Yet by the retaining the muscle you will gain that toned, slither look that is so fashionable in models.

Another important reason why retaining muscle mass is your resting energy expenditure. Your muscles require energy, even when you are not using them intensely. Owing to this, people who retain skeletal muscle burn more calories than people who don't, even if both people are sedentary. Basically being muscular allows you to eat more calories and get away with it!

Muscle mass has also been associated with a general decrease in degenerative diseases as you age (such as diabetes and osteoporosis) as well as lower rates of mental health problems (such as depression and excessive anger).

Overall, the clinical trial performed at the KX fitness center not only supported the notion that the Sirtfood diet can aid weight loss and promote holistic body health, but it also lead to the surprising finding that sirtfoods can retain muscle mass.

Blue Zones

The other evidence for the power of Sirtfoods comes from the 'blue zones'. The blue zones are small regions in the world where people miraculously live longer than everywhere else.

Perhaps most startlingly, you don't just see people live longer in blue zones; you still see them retain energy, vigor and overall health even in their advanced years. Most of us have the fear of becoming decrepit, immobile and overall miserable as we age.

Furthermore, we envision this as starting to occur in our forties and fifties, whilst becoming a fixed reality in our sixties, seventies and eighties. Yet in the blue zones, people not only live past 100 surprisingly regularly, but can walk, work and exercise just as well as those in the younger years. Likewise, they remain mentally slither and don't suffer the cognitive deficits we typically associate with old age.

The blue zones include several areas of the Mediterranean, Japan, Italy and Costa Rica. What do these regions all have in common? They all eat a diet high in sirtfoods. The Mediterranean is famous for its healthy diet involving copious amounts of fish and olive oil. The Japanese savor matcha green tea, whilst the Costa Ricans traditionally indulge in cocoa, coffee and more.

This is the beauty of the sirtfood diet – it isn't trying to make your eating habits artificial and awkward. It is simply copying the healthiest practices that already exist around the world.

17 | P a g .

CHAPTER 2:

The Scientific Basis Of Sirt Diet

There are multiple types and classes of sirtuins that are referred to on the Sirt diet. The first class is generally simply referred to as "sirtuins," which are those found within the human body. However, when sirtuins are found in plants, which are then consumed and can be used by people, they are known as "polyphenols." These polyphenols are organic and bioactive compounds that, while a little different from the sirtuins naturally found within humans, still result in the same biochemical process that results in increased weight loss and promote a variety of health improvements. We will now explore how sirtuins and polyphenols affect the human body and what science has proven about its benefits.

Cellular homeostasis is incredibly important for every aspect of human health. When your cells are in a state of homeostasis, it means that they are working as they should be. They are comfortable, healthy, and doing their job appropriately. They are neither underworking or overworking; everything is as it should be. When you are in cellular homeostasis, you naturally reduce excessive aging or illnesses, instead of promoting whole-body healing and wellness. A 2016 research study by Polish experts on biology, biochemistry, and plant physiology found that sirtuins play a key role in the process of cellular homeostasis, and it shouldn't be underestimated.

Let's go over some of the details of this pioneering study. Don't worry; I will skip the scientific gibberish and speak in layman's terms. Both humans and plants have cellular enzymes that act as a sensor to detect and promote homeostasis. There are different classes of these enzymes, and the third type has been dubbed "sirtuins." Not only are there two different classes of sirtuins, as we mentioned, there are also seven different types.

These types are known simply as Sirt[number 1-7]. Each of these types has one of three roles so that they can all work together throughout the entire body.

One of the roles of some of the sirtuins is to affect the mitochondrial system. This is important, as the mitochondrial system affects a person's weight loss, healing ability, energy levels, and more. Mitochondria are known as a powerhouse. The mitochondrial systems are one of the most important aspects of maintaining homeostasis, as, without it, no human would be able to survive. Those who live with mitochondrial dysfunctions experience severe and widespread symptoms that interfere with daily life. Thankfully, this study found that sirtuins can promote a healthy mitochondrial system leading to cellular homeostasis. In particular, this can help a person increase metabolism and weight loss, reduce inflammation levels, lessen oxidative stress and cellular damage that lead to disease, and promote cellular longevity as you age. As you can imagine, by using sirtuins to activate the mitochondrial system, you not only can help manage and possibly treat mitochondrial disorders, but also other conditions such as obesity, type II diabetes, neurodegenerative diseases, cancer, and more. In part, this positive change is due to the way sirtuins are able to stimulate the mitochondria and mitochondrial proteins to prevent negative changes before they can even occur and treat them directly at the source.

Polyphenols come in a number of classifications with resveratrol and quercetin, being two of them that are more widely known. Each type can have different positive effects, meaning you want to consume sirtuins from a variety of plant-based foods to experience all of the benefits. For instance, you might have heard about resveratrol being found in grape skins and therefore wine, this resveratrol is the very same sirtuins you will be consuming on the Sirt diet. This type of sirtuin specifically has been found to positively affect the Sirt1 category within the body, leading to weight loss, reduced insulin resistance, and improved motor function.

When studying polyphenols, the researchers tracked the number of polyphenols in a given serving for plant matter and their class. For instance, the classes of polyphenols tested include flavanols, flavones, isoflavones, and more. While the researchers in this specific study were unable to test all of the high-sirtuin foods, the ones they did test reinforced what had already been proven: these foods are some of the highest in sirtuin and therefore perfect for the Sirt diet. Some other foods that the researchers proved her high in sirtuins and therefore helpful to consume more of include orange, lemon, grapefruit, eggplant, beans, blackberries, black currants, black grapes, cherries, and rhubarb.

It was also found that other foods and polyphenols can affect each other and how effectively your body absorbs and utilizes them. For instance, if you consume protein (such as meat) and polyphenols together, your body will be unable to absorb either the protein or the polyphenols, as well as it usually would. That is why it is a good idea to drink your green juice separately from your meals. It is still beneficial to add as many Sirtfoods to your meals as possible, even when you are eating protein, but just know that your body will not absorb as many of the sirtuins as it otherwise would. But, if you drink your green juice a couple of hours prior or after you consume protein, you will be able to ensure you get the most benefit out of it possible.

Similarly, the study also found that by heating plants through boiling, steaming, roasting, or cooking in any other way, the sirtuins and their benefits are reduced. Again, this doesn't mean you can't ever cook sirtuin-rich food, but should stay mindful of this and try to eat as many of them raw as possible.

The study concluded that sirtuins are incredibly powerful for general health and wellness, but people should keep in mind how what you consume them with and how you prepare them will affect the sirtuin levels within the food.

When you reduce caloric intake, it results in your metabolic and autophagy processes increasing. However, calorie reduction is not the only way you can experience this benefit, as a study published in Cell Death and Disease in 2010 found. This study found that when you activate your body's natural sirtuins through ingesting polyphenols, you can make use of these same important biological processes, which the researchers could be used to treat cancer in the future. Now, imagine, what if you combine caloric restriction along with increased polyphenol intake? It is likely that by combining these two aspects, both key aspects of the Sirt diet, you could compound the effects for even better results.

By restricting your calories and increasing your Sirt food intake, you can slow down the rate of cellular aging, thereby increasing not only the lifespan of your cells but possibly increase your own life span, as well. Not only that, but as it promotes overall health and wellness, and not simply living to an older age, you might be able to enjoy your golden years happier and healthier, living them to the fullest. Of course, no scientist or doctor, will guarantee you this, and neither will I, as anyone who makes such claims is only making false promises. Yet, I can promise you that science is on the side of Sirtuins and balanced calorie restriction. Study after study has found that both of these elements of the Sirt diet can increase a person's overall health and expected lifespan.

Many people have never heard of the autophagy process, despite its importance. It is a natural biochemical process of the body. Throughout human history, people have unknowingly made use of the autophagy process to help treat disease. They did this largely through fasting. Thankfully, in recent years researchers have learned more about autophagy, not only about its importance but also how we can better make use of it. No longer do we have to fast whenever we want to use this natural reaction, we can use other methods, such as calorie restriction paired with Sirt food intake, to induce it, as well.

The word "autophagy is derived from Latin, with two words combining to translate to "self-eating literally." At first appearance, it may sound like a bad idea to have your body eat itself, but I promise you, in this case, it is something you want to happen. It doesn't hurt you or damages your health. Quite the contrary, if you want to stay healthy, then your body must make use of the autophagy process.

This revolutionary process allows the body to take its damaged and dying cells and recycle them into healthier and younger cells. To put it simply, the autophagy process works similarly to compost. When you are gardening, you get rid of your old useless scraps and molded or rotting produce you are unable to use. But, instead of simply throwing these scraps into the trash, you recycle them into compost to grow new and healthier produce. It is a life cycle that continuously feeds itself so that your garden begins to flourish more day by day, and nothing goes to waste. Your body uses autophagy for the same purpose.

By utilizing the autophagy process, you can help your body to maintain a state of homeostasis, where your cells are consistently being cleaned and repaired. This is especially important in today's day in age when many of us are being assaulted by toxins from every angle. These toxins are in the food we eat, the air we breathe, and the water we drink. Not only are they coming from the outside in, but our own bodies will also produce these toxins when we don't sleep well or make other poor lifestyle choices. Autophagy helps to remove these toxins and reset your body to what it should be.

The main benefits of autophagy include reducing aging and increasing longevity. As the process literally replaces old cells with younger cells, it naturally lessens the rate of aging throughout your entire body and mind. Other benefits include recycling proteins, sorting out and removing toxins that cause neurodegenerative diseases such as Alzheimer's, and increased energy. With all of these benefits, autophagy is currently receiving a lot of attention in the scientific community, as it has a lot of potential in treating some of our most troubling diseases, such as cancer. Many researchers are attempting to find a way to utilize autophagy in the form of a pill to target especially difficult diseases. While this research might still have a long way to go before it is on the market for cancer treatment, in the meantime, you can make use of autophagy in preventing and managing a number of diseases by promoting the process through the Sirt diet. These beneficial effects were well-documented in the 2010 study mentioned.

A study published in 2017 examined why cinnamon is so powerful in improving the insulin response and blood glucose levels, both of which are important for anyone who has diabetes. It is also important for those at a heavier weight, making them predisposed to insulin resistance and high blood sugar. While scientists have long known that cinnamon has a positive effect on this aspect of health, as it has been used for healing ever since ancient times, it has long been a mystery as to why. However, with a new understanding of sirtuins, researchers decided to see if the polyphenol contents within cinnamon were to thank for these powerful healing properties.

CHAPTER 3:

Benefits Of Sirtfoods

Top Sirtfoods incorporate kale, rocket, parsley, red onions, strawberries, pecans, additional virgin olive oil, cocoa, curry flavors, green tea and espresso (indeed, espresso!). As opposed to past advanced diets where the attention is on removing nourishments, with Sirtfoods, the advantages are procured through eating.

In our Sirtfood Diet, preliminary members lost an amazing 7 pounds over the underlying seven days remembering increments for muscle and muscle work. This dramatic impact on fat-consuming, while advancing muscle, is one reason that our Sirtfood-based diet has gotten so well-known with anybody needing to get slender and fit as a fiddle, much the same as the world-class competitors and models. They have supported this way of eating. Alongside fat consuming, Sirtfoods additionally have the one of a kind capacity to usually satisfy a craving, making them the ideal answer for accomplishing a healthy weight and supporting it long haul.

However, to consider it absolutely as a weight reduction diet is to overlook the main issue. This is a diet that has as a lot to do with wellbeing as waistlines. Expanded vitality, brighter skin, feeling alarmed progressively, and better rest is the beautiful 'reactions' from along these lines of eating. Once in a while, the advantages are significantly increasingly momentous, remembering situations where following the diet for the more extended term has turned around metabolic ailments. Such is their health improving impacts that feedbacks demonstrate them to be all the more remarkable then physician recommended tranquillizes in forestalling constant sickness, with benefits in diabetes, coronary illness and Alzheimer's to give some examples. It's no big surprise that it is entrenched that the way of life eating the most Sirtfoods has been the least fatty and healthiest on the planet.

The main concern is evident: If you need to accomplish a progressively vivacious, more slender and healthier body, and establish the frameworks for deep-rooted health and protection from the ailment, at that point, the Sirtfood Diet is for you.

Can you eat meat on Sirtfood?

The diet plan not just incorporates expending a good part of the meat, it suggests that protein be a primary consideration in a Sirtfood-based diet to receive the greatest reward in keeping up digestion and reducing the muscle exhaustion necessary in most diet plans. It is anything but a meat-overwhelming food (we despite everything recall the terrible breath from the Atkins diet), it's in reality very veggie lover well-disposed and caters for practically everybody, which is the thing that makes it so reasonable an alternative.

Leucine is an amino corrosive found in protein, which supplements and improves the activities of Sirtfoods. This implies the ideal approach to eat Sirtfoods is by consolidating them with a chicken breast, steak or another wellspring of leucine, for example, fish or eggs.

Poultry can be eaten uninhibitedly (because it is an excellent wellspring of protein, B nutrients, potassium and phosphorous). That red meat (another fantastic wellspring of protein, iron, zinc and nutrient B12) can be eaten up to multiple times (750g crude weight) seven days.

"Sirtfood" seems like something created by outsiders, brought to earth for human utilization with expectations of picking up mind control and global control. Sirt foods are foods high in sirtuins. Uh, come back once more? Sirtuins are a sort of protein that analyses on organic product flies, and mice have demonstrated direct digestion, increment bulk, and consume fat.

The Sirtfood Diet book was first distributed in the U.K. in 2016. However, during its U.S. arrival in March, has started a greater interest in the arrangement. The eating routine started getting publicity when Adele debuted her slimmer body at the Billboard Music Awards last May. Her coach, Pete Geracimo, is an enormous fanatic of the eating regimen and says the artist shed 30 pounds from following a Sirt food diet. (Here, Adele gets genuine about getting sound.)

As per the manuscript, this arrangement can assist you with consuming fat and lift your vitality, preparing your body for long haul weight reduction achievement and a more drawn out more advantageous, ailment free life. All that while you are drinking red wine. Sounds like virtually the ideal eating regimen, isn't that so? Indeed, before you consume your investment funds loading up on sirtuins-filled fixings, read the upsides and downsides.

How can it work?

At its center, the way to getting in shape is genuinely straightforward: Create a calorie shortfall either by expanding your calorie consume exercises or diminishing your caloric admission. As it may, imagine a scenario where you could skirt the abstaining from excessive food intake and instead activate a "thin quality" without the requirement for extreme calorie limitation. This is the reason of The Sirtfood Diet, composed by nourishment specialists Aidan Goggins and Glen Matten. The best approach to do it, they contend, is Sirt foods.

Sirtfoods are wealthy in supplements that activate an alleged "thin quality" called sirtuin. As indicated by Goggins and Matten, the "thin quality" is activated when a lack of vitality is made after you confine calories. Sirtuins got fascinating to the nourishment world in 2003 when analysts found that resveratrol, a compound found in red wine, had a similar impact on life length as calorie limitation however it was accomplished without lessening admission. (Discover the complete truth about wine and its medical advantages.)

In the 2015 pilot study (directed by Goggins and Matten) testing the adequacy of sirtuins, the 39 members lost a normal of seven pounds in seven days. Those outcomes sound amazing. However, it's critical to understand this is a small example size concentrated over a brief timeframe. Weight reduction specialists additionally have their questions about the grandiose guarantees. "The cases made are extremely theoretical and extrapolate from considers which were, for the most part, centered around basic creatures (like yeast) at the cell level. What occurs at the cell level doesn't mean what occurs in the human body at the full-scale level," says Adrienne Youdim, M.D., the executive of the Center for Weight Loss and Nutrition in Beverly Hills, CA. (Here, look at the best and most exceedingly awful weight control plans to follow this year.)

CHAPTER 4:

What Is The Skinny Gene?

Sirtuins are a kind of protein, which shield the cells in our bodies from getting aggravated through the sickness. However, it has recently demonstrated they can help manage your digestion, the assists in an increment of muscle and consume fat – thus tagging along by its new name 'superfood'.

Sirtuins are a class of proteins that have either mono-ADP-ribosyltransferase or deacetylase action, including deacetylase, desuccinylase, deadenylase, demyristoylase and depalmitoylase movement. The name Sir2 originates from the yeast quality 'quiet mating-type data guideline 2', the quality liable for cell guideline in yeast.

Sirtuins : "Skinny Gene" activator?

Individuals have consistently been entranced with questions about how we can live more and more advantageous lives. Indeed, mainstream researchers have a similar interest with a group of qualities called sirtuins. All of us houses sirtuins—frequently alluded to as our thin qualities—and they are genuinely entrancing, holding the ability to decide things like our capacity to consume fat and remain slim, our powerlessness to infection, and even to what extent we can live.

So what makes sirtuins so incredible? Sirtuins are extraordinary in view of their capacity to change our phones to a sort of endurance mode—setting off a fantastic reusing process that gets out cell waste and consumes fat. The advantages of this are truly astounding: Fat melts away, and we become fitter, more slender, and more beneficial.

So how can we utilize sirtuins?

This brings up the issue: What would we be able to do to actuate sirtuins and receive these astonishing rewards? It is notable that both fasting and exercise enact sirtuins. Be that as it may, oh dear, both interest an unfaltering promise to either food limitation or requesting exercise systems. Reducing calories leaves us feeling exhausted, hungry, and unequivocally irritable, and in the more drawn out term can prompt muscle misfortune and stale digestion. With respect to work out, the sum should have been compelling for weight reduction requires a LOT of exertion. Both can be difficult to achieve.

In 2013, the consequences of one of the most esteemed nourishing examinations at any point completed were distributed. The reason for the evaluation, called PREDIMED, was flawlessly straightforward: It considered the contrast between a Mediterranean-style diet enhanced with either extra-virgin olive oil or nuts and a progressively traditional present-day diet. Results indicated that following five years, coronary illness and diabetes were cut by an extraordinary 30 per cent, alongside significant decreases in the danger of heftiness in the Mediterranean eating regimen gathering. This wasn't unexpected, yet when the examination was explored in more exceptional detail, it was found there was no distinction in calorie, fat, or sugar consumption between the two gatherings. How would you clarify that?

Not every food are made equivalent. Research currently shows that plants contain regular mixes called polyphenols that have enormous advantages for our wellbeing. What's more, when analysts dissecting PREDIMED researched polyphenol utilization among the members, the outcomes were faltering. Over only the five-year time frame, the individuals who expended the most significant levels of polyphenols had 37 per cent fewer passing contrasted with the individuals who ate the least.

Be that as it may, not all polyphenols are equivalent. Information out of Harvard University from more than 124,000 people indicated that certain lone polyphenols were useful for weight control. Thus, an investigation of right around 3,000 twins found that a higher admission of just certain polyphenols was connected with less muscle versus fat and a more beneficial circulation of fat in the body. Polyphenols are without a doubt a shelter for remaining thin and robust, yet in the event that not all polyphenols are equivalent, at that point which is the best? Would it be able to be those that examination has indicated have the capacity to turn on our sirtuin qualities? Exactly the same ones actuated by fasting and exercise?

The pharmaceutical business has rushed to abuse these sirtuin-enacting supplements, contributing many millions to change over them into panacea drugs. For instance, mainstream diabetes tranquillizes metformin originates from a plant and actuates our sirtuin qualities. In any case, as of recently, they have been to a great extent ignored by the universe of nourishment, to the disservice of our wellbeing and our waistlines.

What nutrients activate sirtuins?

With our advantage aroused, we put all the nourishments with the most significant levels of sirtuin-actuating polyphenols together into a different eating regimen. This incorporates extra-virgin olive oil and pecans, the particular considerations in PREDIMED, just as arugula, red onions, strawberries, red wine, dim chocolate, green tea, and espresso among numerous others. At the point when we pilot tried it, the outcomes were shocking. Members shed pounds, while either keeping up or in any event, expanding their bulk. The best part is that individuals detailed inclination extraordinary—overflowing with vitality, resting better, and with remarkable upgrades in their skin.

Thus the Sirtfood Diet was conceived, a progressive better approach to enact sirtuins by eating heavenly nourishments. An eating routine that doesn't include calorie forgetting about, removing carbs, or eating low fat. An eating routine of consideration in which you receive the rewards from eating the nourishments your adoration. The Sirtfood Diet is shaking things up of right dieting guidance and what it truly intends to look and feel incredible. And all from eating our preferred nourishments!

Fasting versus calorie limitation

Supplement hardship or supplement pressure likely incorporates numerous types of dietary limitation, including calorie/dietary limitation, time confined eating regimen (tRD), discontinuous fasting, and fasting. Calorie/dietary limitation depicts the decrease in calorie consumption by generally 20–30%. A period confined eating regimen portrays one supper for each day with typical day by day calorie admission. Intermittent fasting is substituting long periods of standard eating routine and fasting, while unadulterated fasting is finished food starvation for a few backs to back days. In spite of the fact that calorie/dietary limitation has been appeared to influence life expectancy emphatically and disease treatment in research facility settings, interpretation of clinical investigations has been restricted for a few reasons.

In the first place, interminable calorie/dietary limitation has been appeared just to defer the movement of tumor development, and this postpone will happen only for a subset of malignancies likewise, the weight reduction and debilitating of the invulnerable framework made by calorie/dietary limitation makes it hard for disease patients experiencing chemotherapy. On the other hand, a tRD and additionally discontinuous fasting displayed comparative impacts contrasted with calorie/dietary limitation; however, don't bring about weight reduction and can be increasingly mediocre in patients. The main burden for tRD, discontinuous fasting and even calorie/dietary limitation is that they require an all-inclusive time before any insurance produces results that may confine the potential use in malignant growth treatment.

At long last, fasting quickly preceding chemotherapy treatment followed by the arrival to the healthy eating regimen doesn't cause weight reduction in the long haul while possibly upgrading the valuable impacts of chemotherapy. Nonetheless, is it convenient for a malignancy quiet experiencing delayed fasting? Albeit a few examinations have demonstrated that slow starvation is endured in patients with interminable ailment and proposed to be very much taken, it is mentally awkward for some patients. In light of these investigations, it is sensible to suggest that a tRD and additionally discontinuous fasting may accomplish comparative objectives contrasted with calorie/dietary limitation yet with fewer reactions and in that capacity, be increasingly valuable in clinical malignancy treatment, though drawn out fasting might be progressively successful for disease avoidance.

The gainful impacts of fasting have been exhibited for a long time, and all through the typical course of a living being's life, changes in accessible supplements are healthy, and times of starvation are normal. Versatile reactions have created over the life form's advancement to shield it from conceivably deadly threats during these times of famine from any of various potential natural conditions. Numerous past and late investigations have indicated that starvation-actuated pressure opposition is clear and rationed in a wide range of animal types. In both yeast and Escherichia coli, glucose starvation expands assurance against oxidative pressure and, in yeast alone, even a critical increment in life span. Worms and flies have been appeared to profit by the equivalent expanded obstruction against oxidative worry after starvation attributable to the redirection of vitality from cell development to insurance. Various investigations additionally show that fasting ensures the rodent cerebrum, mouse kidney and liver, and human liver from ischemia injury.

Also, starvation or a 10–30% reduction in calorie consumption builds life expectancy up to half and forestalls carcinogenesis in unconstrained, synthetic or radiation-instigated tumorigenesis in a few mammalian test models.

Progressively significant, late investigations further recommend that fasting can crosstalk with sirtuins, a life span quality family, which have been proposed to be essential in maturing and carcinogenesis.

CHAPTER 5:

Sirtfood Diet Phase 1

The sirtfood Diet has two easy to follow phases that last a total of three weeks. After completing the first and second phases you can continue "Sirtifying" your diet by including as many sirtfoods as possible. The idea of sirtifying meals after the first and second phases is to continue on the sirtfood path. It involves incorporating some sirtfood in your favorite dish.

Green juice is a big part of the diet which you have to take one to three times daily.

The sirtfood is designed to be a way of life and not a 'one-time' diet. It recommended that once you complete the first 3 weeks that you continue eating a diet rich in sirtfoods and to continue taking your daily green juice. You can repeat phase 1 and 2 when necessary to have a health boost.

PHASE ONE: HYPER-SUCCESS PHASE

The first phase involves calorie restriction and a lot of green juice and lasts seven days and. This is the first huge step towards losing weight and achieving a slimmer body. It is expected you will lose an average of 7 pounds after completing this phase.

HOW TO FOLLOW PHASE 1

Phase 1 of the Sirtfood Diet includes two distinct stages:

- Stage 1: this is the most intensive and it is during the first 3 days of phase one. Daily Calorie intake is restricted to 1,000 calories. During this stage, you will drink 3 green juice and one main meal (meals rich in sirtfoods).

- Stage 2: on days 4-7 the daily calorie intake increases to 1,500 calories. This includes 2 green fruit juice and two main meals (meals rich in sirtfoods).

You can choose a sirtfood meal from the various recipes as we go along.

There are a few rules to follow when it comes to this diet. The most important thing is to fit it into your lifestyle so it has to achieve a prolonged benefit. However, here are some simple tips to achieve the best impact.

1. Preparation is important: you have to plan to be successful. Get the ingredients and recipes you will need and stock up all you will need, with everything organized and ready the whole process will be easier.

2. Buy a good juicer: the green juice is one of the basic components of this diet and to make it you will need a juicer as a blender will not work. There are several brands of juicer make sure you buy the best and at the same time put your purse in consideration.

3. Save time: if you are the busy type, make sure you prepare cleverly. You can make meals the night before, make juices in bulk and keep in the fridge for up to 3 days but only add the matcha when you are ready to consume it.

4. The earlier the better: late-night eating is not recommended, it is better to eat earlier in the day, do not consume meals and juice after 7 p.m.

5. Space out the Juices: the green juices should be consumed the latest an hour before or two hours before or after a meal and spread out throughout the rather instead of having them too close together.

6. Eat to satisfaction: sirtfood can control the appetite has it has been mentioned, eat until you are satisfied, do not force down the food if you feel satisfied before finishing your meal.

7. Enjoy the process: you do not have to endure the whole process, do not focus on the end goal so it won't feel like a task, and instead stay mindful of the process. This diet is more about celebrating food for all its health benefits and the pleasure and enjoyment it brings. Savor every bite.

Drink it UP

In addition to the recommended daily servings of green juices, you can consume other fluids freely throughout phase 1. Plain water, black coffee, and green tea are recommended. If you have a preference for black or herbal teas, you can include them also. Exclude carbonated drinks, caloric drinks, and fruit juice. You can make it more interesting by adding some strawberries slice or citrus slices to still or sparkling water to make your healthy drink. Keep in the fridge for a couple of hours and you will be amazed to have a refreshing alternative to soft drinks and juices.

It is recommended that your coffee is black, without adding milk because some research shows that the addition of milk to coffee can inhibit or reduce the absorption of the beneficial sirtuin-activating nutrients. Never add milk to your green tea as well as it will have a similar effect. Instead, you can add some lemon juice to your green tea as it increases the absorption of the sirtuin-activating nutrients. The only alcohol accepted for this phase is red wine and it will only serve as a cooking ingredient.

No cause for alarm, this is the hyper-success phase, and you need to be more disciplined but be comforted by the fact that it is only for a week.

The Sirtfood Green Juice

The green juice is an essential part of phase 1. All the ingredients in this juice are powerful sirtfoods, there are several sirtuin-activating nutrients in the juice which make it very potent and able to switch on your sirtuin genes and promote fat loss.

This juice is a must for anyone following the Sirtfood Diet and anyone that wants a bit of health boost. Lemon is also added because of its natural acidity to protect, stabilize, and increase the absorption of the juice's sirtuin-activating nutrients. Touch of apple and ginger can also be added for taste, but they are optional.

Preparation Time: 5 minutes

Cooking Time: 0 minutes

Servings: 1

Ingredients:

30 grams (1 oz) arugula (rocket)

5 grams parsley

2 to 3 large celery stalks including leaves

1 to 2.5cm (0.5 to 1 in) piece of fresh ginger

1/2al of medium size green apple

Juice of 1/2 lemon

½ level teaspoon matcha powder

75 grams (2.5 oz) kale

Directions:

Juice all ingredients except the matcha powder and the lemon.

Add the lemon juice into the green juice.

Pour a small amount of the juice into a glass, add the matcha powder and stir vigorously with a spoon.

It is only when the juice is made and ready to serve that you add the matcha powder.

Once the matcha dissolved add the rest of the juice into the glass and stir again.

You can drink it immediately or save it for future consumption.

Nutrition:

Calories: 104 Cal

Fat: 1.21 g

Carbs: 23.21 g

Protein: 4.69 g

Fiber: 6.1 g

*** For the first stage of phase 1: add the matcha powder only to the first 2 juices of the day.

***for the second stage: add the matcha powder to both juices

The matcha powder is used in the first 2 drinks of the day because it contains a moderate amount of caffeine, for people not used to it, it may keep them awake if taken at night.

CHAPTER 6:

Sirtfood Diet Phase 2

While everyone else has seen these almost always-remarkable modifications ourselves reflection, we know what else you're going to want to see even good outcomes, not just maintain all those advantages. Sirtfoods are, after all, meant to eat for living.

The issue is how you customize what you did in Phase 1 into your daily nutritional routine. This is precisely what inspired us to develop a 14-day maintenance schedule intended to help you make the shift from Phase 1 to your more daily nutritional regimen, thus helping to maintain and expand the advantages of the Sirtfood Diet deeper.

What To Expect

You will maintain the weight loss results through Step 2 and start to lose weight gradually.

Note, the one surprising point we've seen with the Sirtfood Diet is that much or all of the obese people lose is from fat, and many of those definitely contribute some strength in.

Therefore, we would like to inform you again that you don't just evaluate your success by the percentages on measurement. Look into a mirror to see if you look thinner and more muscular, see how well your dress fits, and gobble up the nice comments you'll get from others.

Also remember that as the losing weight continues, so will the medical benefits. By trying to follow the 14-day maintenance program, you are indeed beginning to lay the groundwork for a long-term health for coming years.

How To Follow Phase 2

The trick to progress in this process is having your nutrition packed full of Sirtfoods. To render it as simple as possible, we have prepared a seven-day meal schedule for you to fulfill its requirements, with tasty and healthy recipes, filled with Sirtfoods every day to the rafters. All you have to do is replicate the Seven Day Schedule again to fulfill Step 2's 14 days.

On each of the fourteen days your diet will consist of:

- 3 x balanced Sirtfood-enriched meals

- 1 x Sirtfood green vegetable juice

- 1 to 2 x optional Sirtfood bite snacks

Also, when you've had to eat those, there have been no strict rules. Be agile throughout the day and follow them. Two basic thumb-rules are:

- Have your green vegetable juice either early that morning, at least thirty minutes before dawn meal, or in the middle of the dawn.

- Do your hardest to finish your dinner before 7 p.m.

Portion Sizes

In second phase our attention is not on counting calories. For the common citizen that is not a realistic solution or even an effective one in the lengthy period. Rather we concentrate on healthy servings, quite well-balanced meals, and perhaps most importantly, loading up on Sirtfoods so that you can start to profit from their chubby-burning and health-increasing impact.

Also, we've built the food in the strategy to help satisfy them, which will made you look full and satisfied. That synchronized with Sirtfoods' natural hunger-regulating effects, means you're not going to spend the coming 14 days feeling hungry, but rather generally satisfied, well-fed, and almost well-nourished.

Just like in Phase 1, listen attentively, and be directed by your desire to eat. When you prepare food as per our directions and consider that you are easily full before you have completed a meal, then quit consuming is completely acceptable!

What To Drink

Through most of Step 2 you'll have to have one green vegetable juice daily. This is to maintain you with high Sirtfoods levels.

Much as in Phase 1, you can easily absorb certain fluids in Phase 2. Our favorite beverages comprise remaining plain beer, bottled sweet soda, coffee, and green tea. If black or white tea is your predisposition, please enjoy. The very same holds for black tea. The biggest comment is that throughout Phase 2 you can admire an occasional glass of the red wine. Due to its high content of sirtuin-activating polyphenols, particularly resveratrol and piceatannol, red wine is a sirtfood which makes it by far the right idea of alcoholic drink. But, with liquor itself causing negative impacts on our fat tissue, restraint is always safest, so we suggest restricting the drink to one glass of red wine with a food for 2 to 3 days a week during Phase 2.

Returning To Three Meals

You ingested only one or two meals per day during Phase 1 which allowed you plenty of versatility when you eat your food. Since we are all returning to a more usual schedule and the well-tested practice of 3 meals a day, learning about breakfast is a perfect idea.

Eating nutritious breakfast tends to put us on for the day, rising our amounts of energy and focus. Eating early holds our blood glucose and fat levels in balance, in terms of our metabolism. That meal is a good thing is pointed out by a series of studies usually finding that individuals who eat breakfast often are less probable to obese.

This is because of our body's internal rhythms. Our organs are asking us to feed early in expectation of when we will be much busier and need food. Yet more than a third of us will miss breakfasts on every given day. It's a typical example of our crazy daily life and the feeling that there's just not enough room to eat properly. But as you can see, nothing could be far from the fact with the lovely meals that we have set over here for you. If it's the Sirtfood smoothie that can be drank on the go, the premade Sirt muesli, or the fast and simple Sirtfood scrambled eggs / tofu, having some additional few moments in the morning will yield rewards not only for your whole day but also for your fitness and wellbeing over the lengthy period.

Despite Sirtfoods serving to overcharge our metabolism, there's only more to learn from having a boost from them early that morning to continue your day. It is done not only by eating a Sirtfood-rich meal, but above all by consuming the green vegetable juice, which we suggest you have either first thing every morning — at least 30 minutes before meal — or lane-morning. We get a lot of stories from our own personal experience about people who first sip their green vegetable juice and don't feel thirsty for a few hours afterwards If that is the impact it has on you, waiting a few hours before eating breakfast is well. Just really don't miss this one. Conversely, with a healthy meal, you can start your day, then look for two or three hours to have the green vegetable juice. Be easy, and simply go with anything that soothe for you.

Sirtfood Bites

You should handle it when it relates to eating or leave it. There has been too much discussion over whether eating regular, smaller meals is better for losing the weight, or only sticking to 3 healthy meals a day. The reality is that is not really relevant.

The way we've built the servicing menu for you guarantees you 're going to eat 3 well-balanced Sirtfood-rich meals a day and you might find that you don't always need a snack. So maybe you've been engaged with the kids in the classroom, going out or dashing about and have something to take you until another food. But if that "little thing" will offer you a whammy of Sirtfood vitamins and minerals so wonderful taste, then it's good time. That's why we developed our "Sirtfood Bits." These fun little treats are a truly misery-free treat made completely from sirtfoods: almonds, walnuts, chocolate, turmeric, and extra virgin olive oil and. We suggest eating one, or a possibility of two, every other day for the days that you really need them.

"Sirtifying" Your Meals

We found that the only consistent meals are ones of acceptance, not removal. Yet real achievement goes well beyond that — the diet needs to be consistent with life in modern times. If it's the ease of satisfying the needs of our stressful lifestyle or keeping in with our position at social events as the bon vivant, the way we feed should be trouble-free. You will admire your svelte body and beautiful smile, rather than thinking about the requirements and limitations of kooky products.

What makes Sirtfoods so fabulous is that they are really available, common, and simple to be included in your eating habits. Here, when you cross the distance between step 1 and daily feeding, you can lay the groundwork for a new, enhanced lifelong feeding strategy.

The basic feature is what we call your meal options "Sirtifying." And this is where we take popular meals, along with several classic favorite's, and we retain all the fantastic flavor with some smart swaps and easy Sirtfood additions but add a lot of stuff to that. You'll would see how conveniently this is accomplished all across Phase 2.

Highlights feature our tasty smoothie Sirtfood for the ultimate on-the-go breakfast in a time-consuming universe, and the easy turn from wheat to buckwheat to bring more flavor and bite to a much-loved pasta delicious meal. In the meantime, famous, adored meals such as chili con carne and curry wouldn't even need far more transition, with Sirtfood bonanzas providing local dishes. So, who has said that junk food means bad food? When you start making it yourself, we integrate the accurate lively ingredients of a pizza and erase the culpability. There's no reason to say goodbye to pleasures either, as our soaked pancakes with fruit and dark chocolate pudding has demonstrated. It's not just a cake, it's breakfast and for you it's perfect.

Easy shifts: you keep eating the food that you enjoy when maintaining a good weight and stability. And this is the Sirtfood diet movement

Cooking For More

We accept this, we also are undergoing a time of "Sirtfoods for Everyone," where meals begin, we appeal to many more mouths than one. If it's for friends or family members, the latest meals for supper as well as the Sirtfood-packed soup that we present in this process are planned with everyone in mind. But why not reap the benefits of preparing food batch food to freeze for those still preparing food for one or two to have dishes prepared for this week?

CHAPTER 7:

Sirtfood Diet And Physical Exercise

With 52% of Americans admitting that they think that its simpler to do their charges than to see how to eat steadily, it's fundamental to present a type of eating that turns into a lifestyle as opposed to a coincidental prevailing fashion diet. For a few of us it may not be that difficult to get thinner or hold a solid weight, however the Sirtfood diet can help the individuals who are battling. Be that as it may, shouldn't something be said about joining the Sirtfood diet with work out, is it fitting to stay away from practice totally or present it once you have begun the diet?

The Sirt Diet Principles

With an expected 650 million hefty grown-ups internationally, it's critical to discover smart dieting and exercise systems that are feasible, don't deny you of all that you appreciate, and don't expect you to practice all week. The Sirtfood diet does only that. The thought is that sure nourishments will dynamic the 'thin quality' pathways which are normally actuated by fasting and exercise. Fortunately, certain nourishment and drink, including dull chocolate and red wine, contain synthetic substances called polyphenols that enact the qualities that copy the impacts of activity and fasting.

Exercise during the initial barely any weeks

During the main week or two of the diet where your calorie admission is diminished, it is reasonable to stop or lessen practice while your body adjusts to less calories. Tune in to your body and if you feel exhausted or have less vitality than expected, don't work out. Rather guarantee that you stay concentrated on the rules that apply to a solid lifestyle, for example, including satisfactory day by day levels of fiber, protein and products of the soil.

When the diet turns into a lifestyle

When you do practice it's critical to devour protein in a perfect world an hour after your workout. Protein fixes muscles after exercise, lessens irritation and can help recuperation. There are an assortment of plans which incorporate protein which will be ideal for post-practice utilization, for example, the sirt stew with meat or the turmeric chicken and kale serving of mixed greens. If you need something lighter you could attempt the sirt blueberry smoothie and include some protein powder for included advantage. The kind of wellness you do will be down to you, however workouts at home will permit you to pick when to work out, the sorts of activities that suit you and are short and helpful.

The Sirtfood diet is incredible approach to change your dietary patterns, shed pounds and feel more advantageous. The underlying not many weeks may challenge you yet it's imperative to check which nourishments are ideal to eat and which scrumptious plans suit you. Be benevolent to yourself in the initial barely any weeks while your body adjusts and take practice simple if you decide to do it by any stretch of the imagination. If you are as of now somebody who moderates or extreme exercise then it might be that you can carry on as ordinary, or deal with your wellness as per the adjustment in diet. Similarly, as with any diet and exercise changes, it's about the individual and how far you can propel yourself.

Minerals and nutrients for which ladies may require supplements incorporate calcium, iron, Vitamins B6, B12 and D. Men, be that as it may, need to focus on fiber, magnesium, Vitamins B9, C and E.

That reason applies to weight loss diets also. People's nourishment necessities sway which weight loss diets are increasingly compelling for each sex.

If you're similar to the vast majority, you've seen an astounding number of weight loss projects and patterns go back and forth; practically every one of them have their benefits and practically every one of them work — incidentally. Weight the executives and therapeutic experts fight collectively that the deep rooted, proven blend of good sustenance and ordinary exercise is the most ideal approach to shed pounds and keep it off adequately.

CHAPTER 8:

Top 20 Sirtfoods And Nutrition Tables

Then sirtfood diet comprises of a variety of different foods. The most significant benefit of a sirtfood diet is the wide variety of different food spectrum which can be incorporated in our personalized diet plan. The sirtfood diet can also have coffee and wine, which is the most popular reason that many celebrities are following this diet plan. sirtfoods are the most common and most widely used foods in both the Western and Eastern worlds. To be very specific, sirtfoods are those which contain high levels of a chemical compound called polyphenol. This compound is not uniformly distributed in sirtfoods, but every sirtfood contains specific amounts of polyphenols. You must be thinking that why only polyphenols are being tackled here. The answer is straightforward yet very informative. Polyphenols are the compounds that are present naturally in sirtfood, and many types of research conducted on these foods have confirmed that these foods have the highest impacts when losing extra pounds of fats from the body.

However, the most famous foods in the sirtfood diet are actually twenty in number, and a significant portion of a sirtfood diet comprises of these superfoods. The reason to stick this food on a more significant proportion of the sirtfood diet is the higher number of polyphenols present in these foods, which is essential to unlocking the sirtuin gene in the body. This gene is arguably the most critical gene to trigger many fat loss cycles in the human body. The top twenty sirtfoods are:

1 Arugula

The critical factor is the nutritious benefits provided by this food, which is rich in very unique and rare benefits. It is an outstanding food that can be used in health promotion and anti-aging. It is also called a superfood. A vast scientific literature is dedicated to supporting this food. It contains high amounts of antioxidants, antifungal, antiviral, disinfectant, and protecting benefits. It is also essential In the reduction of cholesterol from the body and thus reduces the chances of atherosclerosis and heart attacks.

A word Rasayana is used in traditional Indian medicine, which is associated with the global benefits of arugula in the human body. Arugula is a natural coolant that can be a protective remedy during hot summers. It also has cooling effects on the liver and stomach.

100g raw arugula	
Calories	25 Cal
Fat	0.66 g
Carbs	3.65 g
Protein	2.58 g
Fiber	1.6 g

2 Buckwheat

Stomach acids, disturbed gut mobility and injured food canal (esophagus) cause heartburn, a condition that affects every human many times in their lives.

Buckwheat prevents heartburn by improving the capacities of the stomach and colon as well as by healing the food canal.

Our large and small intestines have bacteria called E.coli, which are friendly in nature and help in digesting the food.

Buckwheat is helpful to E.coli and thus improves the medium inside the large and small intestine. That helps to prevent irritable bowel syndrome and Crohn's disease, conditions that affect the colon adversely.

It can effectively treat the issues related to constipation due to high concentrations of fiber.

100g buckwheat	
Calories	343 Cal
Fat	3.4 g
Carbs	71.5 g
Protein	13.25 g
Fiber	10 g

3 Capers

The importance of this root plant in traditional Chinese herbalism is well known.

It is considered a great root to promote the self-healing capacity of the body and to maintain vital forces inside the body. Some western herbalists also used this root as the primary source of tonic, which is essential to promote natural immunity and vital capacities of the body.

This root has some fantastic impacts on neural and endocrinal systems of the body. It can be a primary herbal remedy for patients with deficient immunity or those who are treated by chemotherapy and radiotherapy.

These benefits of the herb make it a herbal remedy of choice for cancer patients all over the world. It is a primary adaptive herbal remedy in oncology. Moreover, the use of astragalus is hazard-free and safe.

It has a fantastic impact on bone marrow, and thus, it can easily promote immunity by producing more potent white blood cells that can be used in the war against the deadly pathogens like bacteria and viruses.

It is very high in concentrations of polyphenols, which help in reducing body fats from the body.

100g capers	
Calories	33 Cal
Fat	0 g
Carbs	6.67 g
Protein	3.33 g
Fiber	3.2 g

4 Celery

Much like to buckwheat, celery is very important for our stomach and intestine. Stomach acids, disturbed gut mobility, and injured food canal (esophagus) cause heartburn, a condition that affects every human many times in their lives. Celery prevents heartburn by improving the capacities of the stomach and colon as well as by healing the food canal. Our large and small intestines have bacteria called E.coli, which are friendly in nature and help in digesting the food. Buckwheat is helpful to E.coli and thus improves the medium inside the large and small intestine. That helps to prevent irritable bowel syndrome and Crohn's disease, conditions that affect the colon adversely. It can effectively treat the issues related to constipation due to high concentrations of fiber.

100g raw celery	
Calories	16 Cal
Fat	0.17 g
Carbs	2.97 g
Protein	0.69 g
Fiber	1.6 g

5 Chilies

Chilis are used in both western and eastern foods and can be utilized to achieve higher metabolic rates because these are rich in capsicum.

Capsicum is a potent fat mobilizer that can be used to break adipose tissues into much simpler precursors called fatty acid. Its action is dual.

When these free fatty acids reach in our blood, the action of capsicum in chilies is to increase the basal metabolic rate, which is highly essential to burn these extra fatty acids in the bloodstream and thus promoting a lean physique without extra fat.

100g chilies	
Calories	40 Cal
Fat	0.32 g
Carbs	9.14 g
Protein	1.94 g
Fiber	1.5 g

6 Cocoa

Cocoa is very important for the brain.

By improving overall health and through its antioxidant properties, cocoa can reduce the chances of dementia, Parkinsonism, and much other related pathology.

Fatigue is another crucial aspect to be tackled here. Mental fatigue is related to the exhausting of the brain after prolonged functioning or reduced brain capacities, which can lead to general body pains and low self-esteem.

By providing the nutritional supply to the brain, cocoa can help to prevent the mental as well as general fatigue.

100g cocoa	
Calories	377 Cal
Fat	3 g
Carbs	71.93 g
Protein	15.49 g
Fiber	

7 Coffee

Coffee is the reason for the popularity of the sirtfood diet. This diet regime allows the intake of caffeine in the body so that it can help in breaking the adipose tissues into fatty acid. Coffee, especially caffeine anhydrous, is beneficial in the mobilization of fats. Moreover, coffee also helps in reducing the fatigue in the brain, and it helps in the promotion of mental alertness. It is the biggest cause that the sirtfood diet provides mental focus and alertness to its users, which is not provided in many other ordinary fat loss diet plans.

100g brewed coffee	
Calories	1 Cal
Fat	0.02 g
Carbs	0 g
Protein	0.12 g
Fiber	0 g

8 Extra -Virgin Olive Oil

Olive oil is the most used type of oil throughout the globe. Italian and French diets primarily include olive oils in the main course. Extra virgin olive oil is the lightest form of olive oil. It provides many polyunsaturated fatty acids, which are actually high-density lipids.

These fatty acids are essential in the reduction of blood cholesterol levels as well as they are a vital energy source in the body.

Olive oil is well-researched about its benefits on the brain and cardiac health, and honestly, this attempt is not sufficient to describe the benefits of olive oil.

100g extra virgin coconut oil	
Calories	19 Cal
Fat	0.5 g
Carbs	3.71 g
Protein	0.72 g
Fiber	1.1 g

9 Garlic

For years garlic has been considered one of nature's wonder foods with healing and rejuvenating powers. G

arlic is a powerful antioxidant, antibiotics, and antifungal often used to treat stomach ulcers. It lowers cholesterol by 10 percent and blood pressure by 5 to 7 percent as well as blood sugar levels.

The sirtuin-activating nutrients in garlic are ajoene, myricetin and they are complemented by another key nutrient called the allicin which gives off the characteristic aroma of garlic.

100g raw garlic	
Calories	149 Cal
Fat	05. g
Carbs	33.06 g
Protein	6.36 g
Fiber	2.1 g

10   Green Tea

Green tea is one of the most widely used types of tea around the world because of its health benefits. Green tea is well-researched about its benefits on the brain and cardiac health, and honestly, this writing is not sufficient to describe the benefits of olive oil. Green tea has rich historical importance in Indian ayurvedic medicine as well as in traditional western medicine. It was widely used to promote attention, focus, long-term and short term memory, and brainpower in both children and adults. It was also used as an effective tonic for the heart and vascular health. In some literature, it is also shown that it was also used in lung diseases.

100g green tea	
Calories	1 Cal
Fat	0 g
Carbs	0.3 g
Protein	0 g
Fiber	0 g

11 Kale

Kale is perhaps one of the greatest, healthiest veggies that you can take advantage of—for good reason. It is by far one of the healthiest foods that you can get, and it happens also to be a wonderful source of sirtuins. It may be a bit of an acquired taste, but over time, you can grow to love it—and you will also probably find that it is highly beneficial to your health as well. Eaten on its own, sautéed, as chips, or mixed into a salad, kale is something that you should try to consume regularly. Even better, kale is low in calories while also providing a massive amount of your nutritional value, meaning that you get the best bang for your buck, especially when you are busy restricting calories. One cup of kale, roughly 33 calories, will have over 200% of your daily value of vitamin A, nearly 700% of your vitamin K, 130% of vitamin C, and is loaded up with all sorts of other essentials as well. It also happens to be loaded up with antioxidants like beta-carotene, helping to clear out the body and offering very similar benefits to those that you can expect to see in the Sirtfood Diet.

100g raw kale	
Calories	49 Cal
Fat	0.96 g
Carbs	8.75 g
Protein	4.28 g
Fiber	3.6 g

12   Medjool Dates

The addition of Medjool dates at a listing of foods which spark weight loss and boosts health can come as a surprise--particularly if we inform you that Medjool dates have a staggering 66% glucose. Sugar owns no sirtuin-activating properties at all; instead, it's well-established connections for obesity, cardiovascular disease, and diabetes quite the contrary of that which we're searching to realize. But refined glucose is extremely different from sugar taken in a car supplied by character that's balanced using sirtuin-activating polyphenols: The Medjool date. In full contrast to regular sugar Medjool dates, consumed in moderation, really don't have any real noticeable blood-sugar-raising consequences.

100g medjool dates	
Calories	277 Cal
Fat	0.15 g
Carbs	74.97 g
Protein	1.81 g
Fiber	6.7 g

13   Parsley

Most people do not think of parsley as particularly healthy or even think of it at all when it comes to food just due to the fact that it is not really needed to be consumed on its own. Rather, it is used typically in small amounts as a garnish on food. However, many people are then missing out on all of the wonderful health benefits that parsley has to offcr. It is high in vitamins A, C, and K, and it is also once again, high in antioxidants. You will see this added into the green juice as well.

100g raw parsley	
Calories	36 Cal
Fat	0.79 g
Carbs	6.33 g
Protein	2.97 g
Fiber	3.3 g

14   Red Endive

So far as veggies go, endive is a relatively new kid on the block. Story has it endive was uncovered by accident with a Belgian farmer at 1830. The farmer saved chicory roots, subsequently utilized as a sort of coffee replacement, in his basement, just to forget about them.

Upon his return he found they had sprouted white leaves which upon tasting that he discovered to become tender, crispy, and quite yummy. Today endive is increased all around the Earth, such as the USA, also makes its Sirtfood badge as a result of its remarkable content of this sirtuin activator luteolin. And besides the recognized sirtuin-activating added benefits, luteolin ingestion is getting a promising treatment approach for enhancing sociability in autistic kids. For all those new to endive, it's a crisp feel and a candy favor accompanied with a gentle and agreeable bitterness.

If you are stuck on the best way best to boost endive on your diet plan, you cannot lose by incorporating its leaves into a salad, even in which its own welcome, sour favor provides the ideal snack to some zesty extra virgin olive oil-based dressing. The same as orange, onion is greatest, but the yellowish number may also be regarded as a Sirtfood. Although the red selection can sometimes be more difficult to locate, you may be certain that yellow is a totally appropriate alternate.

100g raw endive	
Calories	17 Cal
Fat	0.2 g
Carbs	3.35 g
Protein	1.25 g
Fiber	3.1 g

15   Red Onions

Onions are a dietary staple as the timing of our ancient predecessors, being among the first crops to be cultivated, some 5,000 decades back.

With such a long history of usage, and these powerful health-giving possessions, onions are admired by many civilizations which have come before us.

The Egyptians maintained them in specific eminence as items of worship, seeing their circle-within-a-circle arrangement as emblematic of eternal life.

Along with the Greeks thought onions fortified athletes. Ahead of the Olympic Games, athletes could consume their way through enormous quantities of onions, drinking the juice! It is an amazing testimony to the way precious early dietary wisdom may be when we believe that onions make their high twenty

Sirtfood standing as they're chock-full of this sirtuin-activating chemical quercetin--that the very chemical the entire world of sports mathematics has lately begun actively exploring and promotion to enhancing sports performance. And red?

Only because they possess the maximum quercetin material, even though the conventional yellow ones do not lag too far away, and also therefore are a fantastic inclusion also.

100g red onions, raw	
Calories	44 Cal
Fat	0.1 g
Carbs	9.93 g
Protein	0.94 g
Fiber	2.2 g

16   Red Wine

Any listing of the best twenty Sirtfoods wouldn't be complete without the addition of red wine, even the most first Sirtfood. From the early 1990s, the French poet made headlines with it had been found that regardless of the French seeming to do anything wrong in regards into health (smoking, lack of practice, and ingestion of rich meals), they'd reduced death rates from cardiovascular disease compared to countries like the United States.

Doctors indicated the reason was that the copious quantities of red wine swallowed. In 1995, Danish researchers released function to demonstrate that low-to-moderate red wine intake reduced death rates, whereas comparable alcohol amounts of alcoholic beverages had no impact and comparable alcohol intakes of hard liquors increased passing prices.

In 2003, obviously, red wine rich material of a bevy of all sirtuin-activating nourishment was discovered, and the remainder, as they say, became background.

But there is more to red wine remarkable résumé. Red wine seems to have the ability to ward off the frequent cold, using average wine drinkers using a higher than 40% decrease in its prevalence. Studies also reveal advantages for oral wellbeing and in avoidance of cavities.

With average ingestion also demonstrated to boost social communicating and out-of-the-box believing, that after-work beverage one of coworkers to talk perform endeavors seems to possess a heritage in powerful science. Naturally, moderation is essential.

Only tiny quantities are required for advantage, and surplus alcohol fast undoes the great.

The sweet spot is apparently sticking over US recommendations up to a single 5-ounce drink every day for women as well as 2 5-ounce beverages every day for men.

To guarantee maximum sirtuin activating bang for the dollar, wines in the New York area (particularly pinot noir, cabernet sauvignon, and merlot) possess the highest polyphenol content of the most frequently accessible wines.

1 glass red wine	
Calories	153 Cal
Fat	0 g
Carbs	4.7 g
Protein	0.126 g
Fiber	0 g

17   Soy

Soy may be somewhat controversial, but it is highly healthy as well, and it will serve as a wonderful plant-based protein for your meals as you read through the recipes that will be provided to you.

You will be able to introduce the plant protein to your diet, meaning that you are getting food that is lower in fats and loaded up with omega-3 and omega-6 fats, which you will need.

100g soy	
Calories	57 Cal
Fat	0.3 g
Carbs	5.59 g
Protein	9.05 g
Fiber	0.7 g

18   Strawberries

Strawberries are another great source of sirtuins that also provide you with a wide range of benefits. Whether you eat them straight without preparing them, include them in a salad, toss them in yogurt, or have any other preferences to how you wish to consume them, there is no doubt about it—strawberries are beneficial. All you have to do is consume them. Strawberries are also high in antioxidants that are great for your heart and blood sugar. They are also quite rich in vitamin C, folate, and manganese. They are deemed a superfood for a reason and they will leave you feeling better than ever.

100g raw strawberries	
Calories	32 Cal
Fat	0.3 g
Carbs	7.68 g
Protein	0.67 g
Fiber	2 g

19   Turmeric

Turmeric pops up repeatedly in all sorts of diets and for a good reason—it is incredibly beneficial to all sorts of people for all sorts of reasons. If you want to add a natural nutritional supplement to your life, this is it. It is highly beneficial to your brain and your body, and even better, it tastes great. Turmeric is full of curcuminoids, antioxidants that can be used to help you keep your body healthy. Turmeric is filled up with this. However, it also aids in inflammation and, therefore, would be able to help with many of the chronic diseases suffered from in the western world. Even better, it boosts the ability of these powers to work by blocking free radicals and then boosting your own antioxidant enzymes to help fight against them. Essentially it is like the backup to the rest of the ingredients while also providing high levels of antioxidants.

Even better, you can throw it together to make delicious curry with many of the other ingredients on this list so far.

100g ground turmeric	
Calories	312 Cal
Fat	3.25 g
Carbs	67.14 g
Protein	9.68 g
Fiber	22.7 g

20   Walnuts

Walnuts are, you guessed it—rich in antioxidants. Even better, however, they also have the addition of omega-3 fatty acids and can help you stay fuller for longer. Whether you will eat handfuls on their own or mix them into anything else, this is a great way for you to help support your body in staying happy and healthy. Most often, these foods are eaten plain, but you can make use of them in all sorts of other contexts, such as in your pasta or cereal, or baking them into something. However, because they are high in fat, you will have to worry about the calorie content if you are eating them during calorie restriction. Be mindful of how many you are eating to ensure that you do not go over them when you are eating.

100g walnuts	
Calories	654 Cal
Fat	65.21 g
Carbs	13.71 g
Protein	15.23 g
Fiber	6.7 g

CHAPTER 9:

Sirtfood Recipes

1 Herby Paleo French Fries With Herbs And Avocado Dip

Preparation Time: 20 minutes

Cooking Time: 35 minutes

Servings: 2

Ingredients:

For the Fries:

1/2 pieces Celery

150 g Sweet potato

1 teaspoon dried oregano

1 / 2 teaspoon Dried basil

1/2 teaspoon Celtic sea salt

1 teaspoon Black pepper

1 1/2 tablespoon Coconut oil (melted)

Baking paper sheet

For the avocado dip

1 piece Avocado

4 tablespoons Olive oil

1 tablespoon Mustard

1 teaspoon Apple cider vinegar

1 tablespoon Honey

2 cloves Garlic (pressed)

1 teaspoon dried oregano

Directions:

Preheat the oven to 205 ° C.

Peel the celery and sweet potatoes.

Cut the celery and sweet potatoes into (thin) French fries.

Place the French fries in a large bowl and mix with the coconut oil and herbs.

Shake the bowl a few times so that the fries are covered with a layer of the oil and herb mixture.

Place the chips in a layer on a baking sheet lined with baking paper or on a grill rack.

Bake for 25-35 minutes (turn over after half the time) until they have a nice golden brown color and are crispy.

For the avocado dip

Puree all ingredients evenly with a hand blender or blender.

Nutrition:

Calories: 146 Cal Fat: 12 g

Carbs: 87.98 g

Protein: 14.51 g

Fiber: 35.8 g

2 Salad With Bacon, Cranberries And Apple

Preparation Time: 10 minutes

Cooking Time: 5 minutes

Servings: 2

Ingredients:

1 hand Arugula

4 slices Bacon

1/2 pieces Apple

2 tablespoon Dried cranberries

1/2 pieces Red onion

1/2 pieces Red bell pepper

1 hand Walnuts

Dressing:

1 teaspoon Mustard yellow

1 teaspoon Honey

3 tablespoon Olive oil

Directions:

Warm a pan over medium heat and fry the bacon until crispy.

Place the bacon on a piece of kitchen roll so that the excess fat is absorbed.

Cut half the red onion into thin rings. Cut the bell pepper into small cubes.

Cut the apple into four pieces and remove the core. Then cut into thin wedges.

Drizzle some lemon juice on the apple wedges so that they do not change color.

Roughly chop walnuts.

Combine the ingredients for the dressing in a bowl. Season with salt and pepper.

Spread the lettuce on a plate / your lunch box and season with red pepper, red onions, apple wedges and walnuts.

Sprinkle the bacon over the salad and divide the cranberries.

Drizzle the dressing over the salad according to taste.

Nutrition:

Calories: 98 Cal

Fat: 82.05 g

Carbs: 50.94 g

Protein: 15.82 g

Fiber: 7.1 g

3 Strawberry Popsicles With Chocolate Dip

Preparation Time: 20 minutes

Cooking Time: 10 minutes plus freezing time

Servings: 5

Ingredients:

125 g Strawberries

80 ml Water

100 g Pure chocolate (> 70% cocoa)

Directions:

Wash the strawberries and slice them into pieces. Puree the strawberries with the water.

If the mixture is not pourable, add some extra water.

Pour the mixture into the popsicle mold and put it in a skewer.

Place the molds in the freezer so the popsicles can freeze hard.

Once the popsicles are frozen hard, you can melt the chocolate in a water bath.

Dip the popsicles in the melted chocolate mixture.

Nutrition:

Calories: 319 Cal

Fat: 1.51 g Carbs: 74.7 g

Protein: 2.94 g

Fiber: 5.1 g

4 Hawaii Salad

Preparation Time: 10 minutes

Cooking Time: 0 minutes

Servings: 2 - 3

Ingredients:

1 hand Arugula

1/2 pieces Red onion

1 piece Winter carrot

2 pieces Pineapple slices

80 g Diced ham

1 pinch Salt

1 pinch Black pepper

Directions:

Slice the red onion into thin half rings.

Remove the peel and hard core from the pineapple and cut the pulp into thin pieces.

Clean the carrot and use a spiralizer to make strings.

Mix rocket and carrot in a bowl. Spread this over a plate / lunch box.

Spread the red onion, pineapple and diced ham over the rocket.

Sprinkle the olive oil and balsamic vinegar on the salad to your taste.

Season with salt and pepper.

Nutrition:

Calories: 198 Cal

Fat: 2.99 g

Carbs: 29.59 g

Protein: 15.47 g

Fiber: 4 g

5 Rainbow Salad For Lunch

Preparation Time: 10 minutes

Cooking Time: 0 minutes

Servings: 2 - 3

Ingredients:

1 hand Salad

1/2 pieces Avocado

1 piece Egg

1/4 pieces green peppers

1/4 pieces Red bell pepper

2 pieces Tomato

1/2 pieces Red onion

4 tablespoons Carrot (grated)

Directions:

Boil the egg as you like. (soft / hard / in between)

Take away the seeds from the peppers and cut the peppers into thin strips.

Cut the tomatoes into small cubes.

Slice the red onion into thin half rings.

Cut the avocado into thin slices.

Cool the egg under running water, peel and cut into slices. Place the salad on a plate / in your lunch box and distribute all the vegetables in colorful rows.

If you feel artistic, you can sort the colors from light to dark. Drizzle the vegetables with olive oil and white wine vinegar. Season with salt and pepper.

Nutrition:

Calories: 158 Cal

Fat: 39.7 g Carbs: 49.64 g

Protein: 17.16 g

Fiber: 20.9 g

6 Strawberry And Coconut Ice Cream

Preparation Time: 15 minutes

Cooking Time: 10 minutes plus freezing time

Servings: 10

Ingredients:

400 ml Coconut milk (can)

1 hand Strawberries

1/2 pieces Lime

3 tablespoons Honey

Directions:

Clean the strawberries and cut them into large pieces.

Grate the lime, 1 teaspoon of lime peel is required. Squeeze the lime.

Put all ingredients in a blender and puree everything evenly.

Pour the mixture into a bowl and put it in the freezer for 1 hour.

Take out the mix out of the freezer and put it in the blender. Mix them well again.

Put the mixture back into the bowl and freeze it until it is hard.

Before serving; Take it out of the freezer about 10 minutes before scooping out the balls.

Nutrition:

Calories: 206 Cal

Fat: 0.07 g

Carbs: 56.54 g

Protein: 24 g

Fiber: 0.45 g

7 Coffee Ice Cream

Preparation Time: 15 minutes

Cooking Time: 10 minutes plus freezing time

Servings: 10

Ingredients:

180 ml Coffee

8 pieces Medjoul dates

400 ml Coconut milk (can)

1 teaspoon Vanilla extract

Directions:

See to it that the coffee has cooled down before using it.

Cut the dates into rough pieces.

Place the dates and coffee in a food processor and mix to an even mass.

Add coconut milk and vanilla and puree evenly.

Pour the mixture into a bowl and put it in the freezer for 1 hour.

Take out the mix out of the freezer and scoop it into the blender.

Pour it back into the bowl and freeze it until it's hard.

When serving; Take it out of the freezer a few minutes before scooping ice cream balls with a spoon.

Nutrition:

Calories: 172 Cal

Fat: 0.22 g

Carbs: 43.15 g

Protein: 1.39 g

Fiber: 4.5 g

8 Banana Dessert

Preparation Time: 15 minutes

Cooking Time: 10 minutes

Servings: 2 - 3

Ingredients:

2 pieces Banana (ripe)

2 tablespoons Pure chocolate (> 70% cocoa)

2 tablespoons Almond leaves

Directions:

Chop the chocolate finely, cut the banana lengthwise, but not completely, as the banana must serve as a casing for the chocolate.

Slightly slide on the banana, spread the finely chopped chocolate and almonds over the bananas.

Fold a kind of boat out of the aluminum foil that supports the banana well, with the cut in the banana facing up.

Place the two packets on the grill and grill them for about 4 minutes until the skin is dark.

Nutrition:

Calories: 232 Cal

Fat: 2.08 g Carbs: 51.3 g

Protein: 2.15 g

Fiber: 2.3 g

9 Salad With Roasted Carrots

Preparation Time: 10 minutes

Cooking Time: 5 minutes

Servings: 2 - 3

Ingredients:

1 hand mixed salad

500 g Carrot

1 piece Orange

100 g Pecans

1/2 teaspoon dried thyme

1 tablespoon Honey

1 tablespoon Olive oil

1 pinch Salt

1 pinch Black pepper

Directions:

Peel the carrots and cut the green. Cut them in half lengthways.

Cook the carrots al dente for 5 minutes and drain well.

Peel the orange and cut it into pieces.

Roughly chop the pecans and briefly fry them in a pan without oil.

Cut the spring onions into thin rings.

Place the carrots in a bowl with 1 tablespoon of olive oil, a pinch of salt and pepper and the thyme.

Roast the carrots briefly on the grill or in a grill pan. Until they have nice grill marks.

Mix the salad with carrots and honey and put on a plate.

Spread the orange slices and pecans over the salad.

Nutrition:

Calories: 108 Cal

Fat: 86.68 g

Carbs: 79.26 g

Protein: 13.93 g

Fiber: 23.8 g

10   Salmon With Capers And Lemon

Preparation Time: 10 minutes

Cooking Time: 15 minutes

Servings: 2 - 3

Ingredients:

2 pieces Salmon fillet

1 tablespoon Coconut oil

2 tablespoon Capers

1/2 pieces

Directions:

Cut the lemon into thin slices.

Take an aluminum tray or piece of aluminum foil that is folded in half.

First lay out 4 slices of lemon and spread the capers on them.

Place the salmon on the capers. Then put a lemon wedge on the salmon.

Fry the salmon on the grill (with aluminum dish / foil).

Season with salt and pepper just before serving.

Nutrition:

Calories: 121 Cal

Fat: 13.75 g

Carbs: 0.84 g

Protein: 0.41 g

Fiber: 0.6 g

11 Pasta Salad

Preparation Time: 15 minutes

Cooking Time: 5 minutes

Servings: 2 - 3

Ingredients:

125 g green asparagus

1 hand Cherry tomatoes

1 / 2 pieces yellow bell pepper

1/2 pieces Red bell pepper

125 g Sesame fusilli

3 tablespoon Olive oil

1 tablespoon Red wine vinegar

1 teaspoon dried oregano

Directions:

Cook the sesame fusilli as indicated on the package.

After cooking the pasta, drain with cold water.

Slice the green asparagus into pieces.

Heat a grill pan and grill the asparagus al dente.

Cut the cherry tomatoes into pieces; some in halves and some in quarters, this gives the salad a nice playful effect.

Cut the two half peppers into long thin strips.

Mix the pasta, asparagus, tomatoes and peppers in a large bowl.

Combine the ingredients for the dressing in a small bowl.

Stir the dressing through the pasta salad.

Nutrition:

Calories: 90 Cal

Fat: 55.75 g

Carbs: 59.33 g

Protein: 55.13 g

Fiber: 4.6 g

12   Pine And Sunflower Seed Rolls

Preparation Time: 20 minutes

Cooking Time: 35 minutes

Servings: 12

Ingredients:

120 g Tapioca flour

1 teaspoon Celtic sea salt

4 tablespoon Coconut flour

120 ml Olive oil

120 ml Water (warm)

1 piece Egg (beaten)

150 g Pine nuts (roasted)

150 g Sunflower seeds (roasted)

Baking paper sheet

Directions:

Preheat the oven to 160 ° C.

Put the pine nuts and sunflower seeds in a small bowl and set aside.

Mix the tapioca with the salt and tablespoons of coconut flour in a large bowl. Pour the olive oil and warm water into the mixture.

Add the egg and mix until you get an even batter. Add 1 tablespoon of coconut flour at a time until it has the desired consistency if the dough is too thin.

Wait a few minutes between each addition of the flour so that it can absorb the moisture. The dough should be soft and sticky.

With a wet tablespoon, take tablespoons of batter to make a roll. Put some tapioca flour on your hands so the dough doesn't stick. Fold the dough with your fingertips instead of rolling it in your palms.

Place the roll in the bowl of pine nuts and sunflower seeds and roll it around until covered. Line a baking sheet with parchment paper. Place the buns on the baking sheet. Cook in the preheated oven for 35 minutes and serve warm.

Nutrition:

Calories: 245 Cal

Fat: 189.53 g Carbs: 159.26 g

Protein: 61.33 g

Fiber: 20.2 g

13 Spiced Burger

Preparation Time: 20 minutes

Cooking Time: 25 minutes

Servings: 2 - 4

Ingredients:

Ground beef 250 g

1 clove Garlic

1 teaspoon dried oregano

1 teaspoon Paprika powder

1 / 2 TL Caraway ground

Toppings:

4 pieces Mushrooms

1 piece Little Gem

1/4 pieces Zucchini

1/2 pieces Red onion

1 piece Tomato

Directions:

Squeeze the clove of garlic.

Mix all the ingredients for the burgers in a bowl. Divide the mixture into two halves and crush the halves into hamburgers.

Place the burgers on a plate and put in the fridge for a while.

Cut the zucchini diagonally into 1 cm slices.

Cut the red onion into half rings. Cut the tomato into thin slices and cut the leaves of the Little Gem salad.

Grill the hamburgers on the grill until they're done.

Place the mushrooms beside the burgers and grill on both sides until cooked but firm.

Place the zucchini slices beside it and grill briefly.

Now it's time to build the burger!

Place 2 mushrooms on a plate, then stack the lettuce, a few slices of zucchini and tomatoes. Then put the burger on top and finally add the red onion.

Nutrition:

Calories: 122 Cal

Fat: 1.52 g

Carbs: 25.57 g

Protein: 6.17 g

Fiber: 7.3 g

14 Chicken Skewers With Cashew Sauce

Preparation Time: 25 minutes

Cooking Time: 30 minutes

Servings: 3

Ingredients:

2 pieces Chicken legs

1 1 / 2 EL Coconut amino

1 clove Garlic

1 tablespoon Sesame seeds

1 tablespoon Olive oil

1/2 pieces Spring onions

4 pieces Toothpicks

Cashew Sauce:

75 g unsalted cashew nuts

75 ml Coconut milk

1 1 / 2 EL Coconut amino

1 clove Garlic

Directions:

Cut the chicken legs into cubes and put them in a bowl. Add coconut amino and olive oil and press the clove of garlic into the mixture.

Stir with a spoon and let marinate for about 30 minutes.

In the meantime, put a few long wooden skewers in water.

Put the chicken cubes on the skewers.

Put the ingredients for the cashew sauce in a food processor and grind until you get a smooth sauce.

Place the sauce in a saucepan and heat slowly until hot. (slow is very important, otherwise the sauce can separate)

Cut the spring onions into rings.

Grill the chicken skewers on the grill, garnish with the spring onions and sesame seeds. Serve with the warm cashew sauce.

Nutrition:

Calories: 219 Cal

Fat: 85.54 g

Carbs: 29 g

Protein: 15 g

Fiber: 58 g

15 Vegetable Skewers

Preparation Time: 10 minutes

Cooking Time: 10 minutes

Servings: 5

Ingredients:

1/2 pieces Eggplant

1/2 pieces Zucchini

1 / 2 pieces yellow bell pepper

4 pieces Cherry tomatoes

1 clove Garlic

3 tablespoons Olive oil

1 1 / 2 EL Balsamic vinegar

4 pieces Toothpicks

Directions:

Place the skewers in a bowl or bowl of water about half an hour before you start cooking

Cut the aubergine, zucchini and bell pepper into 8 pieces.

Put all the vegetables on the skewers.

Squeeze the garlic and mix with the oil and balsamic vinegar.

Drizzle the dressing over the skewers.

Grill the vegetables on the grill for about 5 minutes.

Drizzle a little more dressing on the skewers before serving.

Nutrition:

Calories: 571 Cal

Fat: 42.28 g

Carbs: 48.82 g

Protein: 9.18 g

Fiber: 19.8 g

16 Pork Chops With Orange And Mustard Glaze

Preparation Time: 30 minutes

Cooking Time: 45 minutes

Servings: 4

Ingredients:

2 pieces Rib cutlet

1 piece Orange

THE SIRTFOOD DIET

1 tablespoon Mustard yellow

1 tablespoon Olive oil

2 sprigs fresh rosemary

Directions:

Put the pork chops in a bowl.

Squeeze the orange and put it in a bowl with the mustard and olive oil.

Take the rosemary leaves and add them to the orange mixture.

Beat well for a minute and then pour the mixture over the pork chops.

Leave on for at least 45 minutes.

Grill the pork chops on the grill.

Nutrition:

Calories: 230 Cal

Fat: 36.24 g

Carbs: 0.91 g

Protein: 82.38 g

Fiber: 0.6 g

17 Grilled Sweet Potato With Coriander Dressing

Preparation Time: 10 minutes

Cooking Time: 15 minutes

Servings: 3

Ingredients:

2 pieces Sweet potato

1 tablespoon Coconut oil

Dressing:

1 hand fresh coriander

2 1/2 tablespoon Olive oil (mild)

1 tablespoon Natural vinegar

1/2 pieces Red pepper

Directions:

Wash the sweet potato and cut lengthways into slices about 1 cm thick.

Place the slices in a bowl and pour coconut oil over them. Add a little salt and mix well.

Grill the sweet potato on the grill until it is done.

In the meantime, do the dressing; Put all the ingredients in the food processor and mix to an even dressing.

Serve the sweet potato with the dressing.

Nutrition:

Calories: 220 Cal

Fat: 48.12 g

Carbs: 71.82 g

Protein: 2.77 g

Fiber: 5.1 g

18 Sweet Potato Salad With Bacon

Preparation Time: 15 minutes

Cooking Time: 30 minutes

Servings: 4

Ingredients:

Five slices of bacon

Sweet potato (peeled and diced)

Garlic clove (squeezed)

A spoonful of lemon juice

A spoon of olive oil

Balsamic vinegar preparation spoon

Directions:

Preheat the oven to 220 ° C and cover the pan with parchment paper.

Place the bacon on the baking sheet and cook until crispy (about 20 minutes).

Remove the bacon from the pan, crisp and mince.

Mix the sweet potato cubes with garlic in the same pot, season with a little olive oil, and fry in the oven for about 30 minutes.

Season olive oil, vinegar and lime juice in a bowl.

Remove the French fries from the oven, mix with bacon French fries, and season with spices.

If necessary, add rockets and pine nuts at the end.

Nutrition:

Calories: 405 Cal

Fat: 10.67 g

Protein: 11.07 g

Sugar: 4.33 g

19 Salad With Melon And IIam

Preparation Time: 20 minutes

Cooking Time: 20 minutes

Servings: 4

Ingredients:

5 slices Bacon

2 pieces Sweet potato (peeled and diced)

3 cloves Garlic (pressed)

4 tablespoon Lime juice

3 tablespoon Olive oil

1 tablespoon Balsamic vinegar

Directions:

Preheat the oven to 220 ° C and cover a baking sheet with parchment paper.

Place the bacon on the baking sheet and bake until crispy in the oven (approx. 20 minutes).

Take the bacon off the baking sheet, let it cool and chop it.

Mix the sweet potato cubes with garlic on the same baking sheet, drizzle with a little mild olive oil and fry them in the oven for about 30 minutes.

Prepare a dressing made from olive oil, vinegar, and lime juice by mixing them in a bowl.

Take the potato cubes out of the oven, mix them with the bacon pieces and drizzle them with the dressing.

If you like, add rocket and/or pine nuts at the end.

Nutrition:

Calories: 127 Cal

Fat: 99.07 g

Carbs: 79.33 g

Protein: 19.06 g

Fiber: 4.8 g

20 Paleo Chicken Wraps

Preparation Time: 15 minutes

Cooking Time: 15 minutes

Servings: 2

Ingredients:

2 pieces Egg

240 ml Almond milk

1 teaspoon Olive oil (mild)

1 / 4 TL Celtic sea salt

75 g Tapioca flour

Coconut flour3 tablespoon

Chicken breast10 slices

Directions:

Whisk the eggs in a container, then add almond milk, olive oil, and salt.

Add tapioca and coconut flour and stir with a whisk until you get an even batter.

Grease a pan and pour 1/6 of the batter into the pan.

The wraps should have a diameter of approx. 15 cm.

Fry the wraps on both sides until golden brown.

Repeat this step with the rest of the dough.

Fill the wraps with chicken and possibly additional salad or raw vegetables as you like.

Nutrition:

Calories: 256 Cal

Fat: 92.16 g Carbs: 70.22 g

Protein: 62 g

Fiber: 1.2 g

21   Chocolate Breakfast Muffins

Preparation Time: 15 minutes

Cooking Time: 15 minutes

Servings: 8

Ingredients:

250 g Almond paste

3 pieces Banana (ripe)

2 pieces Egg

1 teaspoon Vanilla extract

1/2 teaspoon Tartar baking powder

100 g Chocolate chips

Directions:

Preheat the oven to 200 ° C and prepare a baking sheet with paper or silicone muffin tins.

Place all ingredients (except the optional chocolate chips) in a food processor and mix them into a smooth, sticky dough.

Optional: add pieces of chocolate and stir

Optional: add pieces of chocolate and stir

Put the dough in the muffin tins and bake until golden brown and cooked in about 12-15 minutes.

Nutrition:

Calories: 200 Cal

Fat: 145.26 g

Carbs: 123.88 g

Protein: 72.92 g

Fiber: 34 g

22 Apple Cinnamon Wraps

Preparation Time: 20 minutes

Cooking Time: 20 minutes

Servings: 5

Ingredients:

For the wraps:

2 pieces Egg (beaten)

240 ml Almond milk

1 teaspoon Olive oil (mild)

1 / 4 TL Celtic sea salt

75 g Tapioca flour

3 tablespoons Coconut flour

For garnish:

1 tablespoon Ghee

1 piece Apple

1 teaspoon Cinnamon

1 hand Cranberries

1 teaspoon Lemon juice

Directions:

Whisk the eggs in a container, then add almond milk, olive oil, and salt.

Add the tapioca and coconut flour and stir with a whisk until you get an even batter. Grease a pan and pour 1/6 of the batter into the pan. The wraps should have a diameter of approx. 15 cm.

Fry the wraps on both sides until golden brown.

Heat the ghee in a pan.

Add the diced apple, cinnamon, cranberries and lemon juice and cook over medium heat until the apple is soft. Spoon the apple onto the wrap and fold it into a roll.

Enjoy it!

Nutrition:

Calories: 278 Cal

Fat: 24.24 g Carbs: 97.8 g

Protein: 19 g Fiber: 6.9 g

23   Avocado And Salmon Salad Buffet

Preparation Time: 10 minutes

Cooking Time: 10 minutes

Servings: 2 - 3

Ingredients:

1/2 pieces Cucumber

1 piece Avocado

1/2 pieces Red onion

250 g mixed salad

4 slices smoked salmon

Directions:

Slice the cucumber and avocado into cubes and chop the onion.

Spread the lettuce leaves on deep plates and spread the cucumber, avocado, and onion over the lettuce. Season with salt and pepper (you can also add a little olive oil to the salad). Place smoked salmon slices on top and serve.

Nutrition:

Calories: 209 Cal

Fat: 21 g

Carbs: 33.19 g

Protein: 8.82 g

Fiber: 16.7 g

24   Paleo-Force Bars

Preparation Time: 15 minutes

Cooking Time: 10 minutes plus freezing time

Servings: 10

Ingredients:

10 pieces Medjoul dates (cored)

100 g Grated coconut

100 g crushed linseed

75 g Cashew nuts

60 g Coconut oil

Directions:

Put all ingredients in a food processor and pulse until a sticky and granular dough is formed.

Line a small baking sheet with parchment paper.

Spread the mixture on the bottom of the baking sheet and press down firmly.

Let them solidify and harden them in the freezer for a few hours.

After the mixture has hardened, cut it into bars.

If you want to pack them as individual snacks, wrap the bars in cling film or baking paper.

Nutrition:

Calories: 267 Cal

Fat: 33.76 g

Carbs: 89.14 g

Protein: 18.2 g

Fiber: 11.8 g

25   Vinaigrette

Preparation Time: 5 minutes

Cooking Time: 0 minutes

Servings: 1 cup

Ingredients:

4 teaspoons Mustard yellow

4 tablespoon White wine vinegar

1 teaspoon Honey

165 ml Olive oil

Directions:

Whisk the mustard, vinegar, and honey in a bowl with a whisk until they are well mixed.

Add the olive oil in small amounts while whisking with a whisk until the vinaigrette is thick.

Season with salt and pepper.

Nutrition:

Calories: 45 Cal

Fat: 0.67 g

Carbs: 7.18 g

Protein: 0.79 g

Fiber: 0.8 g

26   Spicy Ras-El-Hanout Dressing

Preparation Time: 10 minutes

Cooking Time: 5 minutes

Servings: 1 cup

Ingredients:

125 ml Olive oil

1 piece Lemon (the juice)

2 teaspoons Honey

1 ½ teaspoons Ras el Hanout

½ pieces Red pepper

Directions:

Remove the seeds from the chili pepper.

Chop the chili pepper as finely as possible.

Place the pepper in a bowl with lemon juice, honey, and Ras-El-Hanout and whisk with a whisk.

Then add the olive oil drop by drop while continuing to whisk.

Nutrition:

Calories: 81 Cal

Fat: 0.86 g

Carbs: 20.02 g

Protein: 1.32 g

Fiber: 0.9 g

27 Chicken Rolls With Pesto

Preparation Time: 15 minutes

Cooking Time: 20 minutes

Servings: 4

Ingredients:

2 tablespoon Pine nuts

25 g Yeast flakes

1 clove Garlic (chopped)

15 g fresh basil

85 ml Olive oil

2 pieces Chicken breast

Directions:

Preheat the oven to 175 ° C.

Bake the pine nuts in a dry pan over medium heat for 3 minutes until golden brown. Place on a plate and set aside.

Put the pine nuts, yeast flakes and garlic in a food processor and grind them finely.

Add the basil and oil and mix briefly until you get a pesto.

Season with salt and pepper.

Place each piece of chicken breast between 2 pieces of cling film

Beat with a saucepan or rolling pin until the chicken breast is about 0.6 cm thick.

Remove the cling film and spread the pesto on the chicken.

Roll up the chicken breasts and use cocktail skewers to hold them together.

Season with salt and pepper.

Melt the coconut oil in a saucepan and brown the chicken rolls over high heat on all sides.

Put the chicken rolls in a baking dish, place in the oven and bake for 15-20 minutes until they are done.

Slice the rolls diagonally and serve with the rest of the pesto.

Goes well with a tomato salad.

Nutrition:

Calories: 105 Cal

Fat: 54.19 g

Carbs: 6.53 g

Protein: 127 g

Fiber: 1.9 g

28   Mustard

Preparation Time: 15 minutes

Cooking Time: 5 minutes plus chilling time

Servings: 1 cup

Ingredients: 60 ml Water

60 g Mustard seeds

60 ml Apple cider vinegar

2 teaspoons Lemon juice

90 g Honey

1/2 teaspoon dried turmeric

Directions: Put mustard seeds, water and vinegar in a glass, close well and leave in the fridge for 12 hours. Put all ingredients in a tall measuring cup the following day. Use your hand blender to puree everything. Try the mustard and add some honey or salt. Store the mustard in a clean glass in the fridge, it will keep for at least 3 weeks.

Nutrition:

Calories: 280 Cal

Fat: 21.87 g Carbs: 93.73 g

Protein: 16.24 g Fiber: 8.2 g

29 Vegetarian Curry From The Crock Pot

Preparation time: 6 hours 10 minutes

Cooking time: 6 hours

Servings: 2

Ingredients:

4 pieces Carrot

2 pieces Sweet potato

1 piece Onion

3 cloves Garlic

2 tablespoon Curry powder

1 teaspoon Ground caraway (ground)

¼ teaspoon Chili powder

1/4 TL Celtic sea salt

1 pinch Cinnamon

100 ml Vegetable broth

400 g Tomato cubes (can)

250 g Sweet peas

tablespoon Tapioca flour

Directions:

Roughly chop vegetables and potatoes and press garlic.

Halve the sugar snap peas.

Put the carrots, sweet potatoes and onions in the slow cooker.

Mix tapioca flour with curry powder, cumin, chili powder, salt and cinnamon and sprinkle this mixture on the vegetables.

Pour the vegetable broth over it.

Close the lid of the slow cooker and let it simmer for 6 hours on a low setting.

Stir in the tomatoes and sugar snap peas for the last hour.

Cauliflower rice is a great addition to this dish.

Nutrition:

Calories: 397 kcal

Protein: 9.35 g

Fat: 6.07 g

Carbohydrates: 81.55 g

30 Fried Cauliflower Rice

Preparation Time: 20 minutes

Cooking Time: 25 minutes

Servings: 4

Ingredients:

1 piece Cauliflower

2 tablespoon Coconut oil

1 piece Red onion

4 cloves Garlic

60 ml Vegetable broth

1.5 cm fresh ginger

1 teaspoon Chili flakes

½ pieces Carrot

½ pieces Red bell pepper

½ pieces Lemon (the juice)

2 tablespoon Pumpkin seeds

2 tablespoon fresh coriander

Directions:

Cut the cauliflower into small rice grains in a food processor.

Finely chop the onion, garlic and ginger, cut the carrot into thin strips, dice the bell pepper and finely chop the herbs.

Melt 1 tablespoon of coconut oil in a pan and add half of the onion and garlic to the pan and fry briefly until translucent.

Add cauliflower rice and season with salt. Pour in the broth and stir everything until it evaporates and the cauliflower rice is tender.

Take the rice out of the pan and set it aside. Melt the rest of the coconut oil in the pan and add the remaining onions, garlic, ginger, carrots and peppers.

Fry for a few minutes until the vegetables are tender. Season them with a little salt. Add the cauliflower rice again, heat the whole dish and add the lemon juice.

Garnish with pumpkin seeds and coriander before serving.

Nutrition:

Calories: 261 Cal

Fat: 35.61 g Carbs: 34.5 g

Protein: 10.27 g Fiber: 8.4 g

31 Mediterranean Paleo Pizza

Preparation Time: 15 minutes

Cooking Time: 15 minutes

Servings: 3 - 4

Ingredients:

For the pizza crusts:

120 g Tapioca flour

1 teaspoon Celtic sea salt

2 tablespoon Italian spice mix

45 g Coconut flour

120 ml Olive oil (mild)

Water (warm) 120 ml

Egg (beaten) 1 piece

For covering:

2 tablespoon Tomato paste (can)

½ pieces Zucchini

½ pieces Eggplant

2 pieces Tomato

2 tablespoon Olive oil (mild)

1 tablespoon Balsamic vinegar

Directions:

Preheat the oven to 190 ° C and line a baking sheet with parchment paper.

Cut the vegetables into thin slices.

Mix the tapioca flour with salt, Italian herbs and coconut flour in a large bowl.

Pour in olive oil and warm water and stir well.

Then add the egg and stir until you get an even dough.

If the dough is too shrill, add 1 tablespoon of coconut flour at a time until it is the desired thickness. Always wait a few minutes before adding more coconut flour, as it will take some time to absorb the moisture. The intent is to get a soft, sticky dough.

Split the dough into two parts and spread them in flat circles on the baking sheet (or make 1 large sheet of pizza as shown in the picture).

Bake in the oven for about 10 minutes.

Brush the pizza with tomato paste and spread the aubergines, zucchini and tomato overlapping on the pizza.

Drizzle the pizza with olive oil and bake in the oven for another 10-15 minutes.

Drizzle balsamic vinegar over the pizza before serving.

Nutrition:

Calories: 229 Cal

Fat: 103 g Carbs: 32 g

Protein: 24 g Fiber: 31 g

32   Fried Chicken And Broccolini

Preparation Time: 10 minutes

Cooking Time: 15 minutes

Servings: 5

Ingredients:

2 tablespoon Coconut oil

400 g Chicken breast

Bacon cubes 150 g

Broccolini 250 g

Directions:

Cut the chicken into cubes.

Melt the coconut oil in a pan over medium heat and brown the chicken with the bacon cubes and cook through.

Season with chili flakes, salt and pepper.

Add broccolini and fry.

Stack on a plate and enjoy!

Nutrition:

Calories: 198 Cal

Fat: 64.2 g Carbs: 0 g

Protein: 83.4 g Fiber: 0 g

33   Braised Leek With Pine Nuts

Preparation Time: 15 minutes

Cooking Time: 15 minutes

Servings: 4

Ingredients:

20 g Ghee

2 teaspoon Olive oil

2 pieces Leek

150 ml Vegetable broth

fresh parsley

1 tablespoon fresh oregano

1 tablespoon Pine nuts (roasted)

Directions:

Cut the leek into thin rings and finely chop the herbs. Roast the pine nuts in a dry pan over medium heat.

Melt the ghee together with the olive oil in a large pan.

Cook the leek until golden brown for 5 minutes, stirring constantly.

Add the vegetable broth and cook for another 10 minutes until the leek is tender.

Stir in the herbs and sprinkle the pine nuts on the dish just before serving.

Nutrition:

Calories: 189 Cal

Fat: 9.67 g

Carbs: 25.21 g

Protein: 2.7 g

Fiber: 3.2 g

34 Sweet And Sour Pan With Cashew Nuts

Preparation Time: 15 minutes

Cooking Time: 20 minutes

Servings: 4

Ingredients:

2 tablespoon Coconut oil

2 pieces Red onion

2 pieces yellow bell pepper

250 g White cabbage

150 g Pak choi

50 g Mung bean sprouts

4 pieces Pineapple slices

50 g Cashew nuts

For the sweet and sour sauce:

60 ml Apple cider vinegar

4 tablespoon Coconut blossom sugar

1½ tablespoon Tomato paste

1 teaspoon Coconut-Aminos

2 teaspoon Arrowroot powder

75 ml Water

Directions:

Roughly cut the vegetables.

Mix the arrow root with five tablespoons of cold water into a paste.

Then mix in all the other ingredients for the sauce in a saucepan and add the arrowroot paste for binding.

Melt the coconut oil in a pan and fry the onion.

Add the bell pepper, cabbage, Pak choi and bean sprouts and stir-fry until the vegetables become a little softer.

Add the pineapple and cashew nuts and stir a few more times.

Pour a little sauce over the wok dish and serve.

Nutrition:

Calories: 114 Cal

Fat: 55.62 g

Carbs: 55.3 g

Protein: 30.49 g

Fiber: 24.1 g

35 Casserole With Spinach And Eggplant

Preparation Time: 30 minutes

Cooking Time: 40 minutes

Servings: 4

Ingredients:

1-piece Eggplant

2 pieces Onion

Olive oil 3 tablespoon

Spinach (fresh) 450 g

Tomatoes 4 pieces

Egg 2 pieces

60 ml Almond milk

2 teaspoons Lemon juice

4 tablespoon Almond flour

Directions:

Preheat the oven to 200 ° C.

Cut the eggplants, onions and tomatoes into slices and sprinkle salt on the eggplant slices.

Brush the eggplants and onions with olive oil and fry them in a grill pan.

Shrink the spinach in a large saucepan over moderate heat and drain in a sieve.

Put the vegetables in layers in a greased baking dish: first the eggplant, then the spinach and then the onion and the tomato. Repeat this again.

Whisk eggs with almond milk, lemon juice, salt and pepper and pour over the vegetables.

Sprinkle almond flour over the dish and bake in the oven for about 30 to 40 minutes.

Nutrition:

Calories: 89 Cal

Fat: 63.64 g

Carbs: 61 g

Protein: 27.9 g

Fiber: 21.8 g

36   Vegetarian Paleo Ratatouille

Preparation Time: 45 minutes

Cooking Time: 55 minutes

Servings: 4

Ingredients:

200 g Tomato cubes (can)

1/2 pieces Onion

2 cloves Garlic

1/4 teaspoon dried oregano

1 / 4 TL Chili flakes

2 tablespoon Olive oil

1 piece Eggplant

1 piece Zucchini

1 piece hot peppers

1 teaspoon dried thyme

Directions:

Preheat the oven to 180 ° C and lightly oil a round or oval shape.

Finely chop the onion and garlic.

Mix the tomato cubes with garlic, onion, oregano and chili flakes, season with salt and pepper and put on the bottom of the baking dish.

Use a mandolin, a cheese slicer or a sharp knife to cut the eggplant, zucchini and hot pepper into very thin slices.

Put the vegetables in a bowl (make circles, start at the edge and work inside).

Drizzle the remaining olive oil on the vegetables and sprinkle with thyme, salt and pepper.

Cover the baking dish with a piece of parchment paper and bake in the oven for 45 to 55 minutes.

Enjoy it!

Nutrition:

Calories: 156 Cal

Fat: 28.97 g

Carbs: 71.62 g

Protein: 11.31 g

Fiber: 24.7 g

37   Courgette And Broccoli Soup

Preparation Time: 10 minutes

Cooking Time: 15 minutes

Servings: 4

Ingredients:

2 tablespoon Coconut oil

1 piece Red onion

2 cloves Garlic

300 g Broccoli

1 piece Zucchini

750 ml Vegetable broth

Directions:

Finely cut the onion and garlic, cut the broccoli into florets and the zucchini into slices.

Melt the coconut oil in a soup pot and fry the onion with the garlic.

Cook the zucchini for a few minutes.

Add broccoli and vegetable broth and simmer for about 5 minutes.

Puree the soup with a hand blender and season with salt and pepper.

Nutrition:

Calories: 356 Cal

Fat: 28.85 g

Carbs: 21.15 g

Protein: 11.4 g

Fiber: 10.2 g

38 Frittata With Spring Onions And Asparagus

Preparation Time: 25 minutes

Cooking Time: 30 minutes

Servings: 8

Ingredients:

5 pieces Egg

80 ml Almond milk

2 tablespoon Coconut oil

1 clove Garlic

100 g Asparagus tips

4 pieces Spring onions

1 teaspoon Tarragon

1 pinch Chili flakes

Directions:

Preheat the oven to 220 ° C.

Squeeze the garlic and finely chop the spring onions.

Whisk the eggs with the almond milk and season with salt and pepper.

Melt 1 tablespoon of coconut oil in a medium-sized cast iron pan and briefly fry the onion and garlic with the asparagus.

Remove the vegetables from the pan and melt the remaining coconut oil in the pan.

Pour in the egg mixture and half of the entire vegetable.

Place the pan in the oven for 15 minutes until the egg has solidified.

Then take the pan out of the oven and pour the rest of the egg with the vegetables into the pan.

Place the pan in the oven again for 15 minutes until the egg is nice and loose.

Sprinkle the tarragon and chili flakes on the dish before serving.

Nutrition:

Calories: 297Cal

Fat: 75.69 g

Carbs: 14.65 g

Protein: 48.46 g

Fiber: 3.8 g

39 Cucumber Salad With Lime And Coriander

Preparation Time: 10 minutes

Cooking Time: 0 minutes

Servings: 3

Ingredients:

1 piece Red onion

2 pieces Cucumber

2 pieces Lime (juice)

2 tablespoon fresh coriander

Directions:

Cut the onion into rings and thinly slice the cucumber. Chop the coriander finely.

Place the onion rings in a bowl and season with about half a tablespoon of salt.

Rub it in well and then fill the bowl with water.

Pour off the water and then rinse the onion rings thoroughly (in a sieve).

Put the cucumber slices together with onion, lime juice, coriander and olive oil in a salad bowl and stir everything well.

Season with a little salt.

You can put aside this dish in the refrigerator in a covered bowl for a few days.

Nutrition:

Calories: 115 Cal

Fat: 0.83 g

Carbs: 26.44 g

Protein: 3.99 g

Fiber: 5.1 g

40 Mexican Bell Pepper Filled With Egg

Preparation Time: 15 minutes

Cooking Time: 15 minutes

Servings: 3

Ingredients:

1 tablespoon Coconut oil

4 pieces Egg

1 piece Tomato

1 pinch Chili flakes

1/4 teaspoon Ground cumin

¼ teaspoon Paprika powder

½ pieces Avocado

1 piece green peppers

2 tablespoon fresh coriander

Directions:

Cut the tomatoes and avocado into cubes and finely chop the fresh coriander.

Melt the coconut oil in a pan over medium heat, beat the eggs in the pan and add the tomato cubes.

Keep stirring until the eggs solidify and season with chili, caraway, paprika, pepper, and salt.

Finally add the avocado.

Place the egg mixture in the pepper halves and garnish with fresh coriander.

Nutrition:

Calories: 195 Cal

Fat: 82.55 g

Carbs: 28.82 g

Protein: 41.81 g

Fiber: 15.5 g

41 Honey Mustard Dressing

Preparation Time: 5 minutes

Cooking Time: 0 minutes

Servings: 1 cup

Ingredients:

4 tablespoon Olive oil

11/2 teaspoon Honey

11/2 teaspoon Mustard

1 teaspoon Lemon juice

1 pinch Salt

Directions:

Mix olive oil, honey, mustard and lemon juice into an even dressing with a whisk.

Season with salt.

Nutrition:

Calories: 218 Cal

Fat: 54.93 g

Carbs: 33.93 g

Protein: 1.16 g

Fiber: 1.2 g

42 Paleo Chocolate Wraps With Fruits

Preparation time: 25 minutes

Cooking time: 0 minutes

Servings: 2

Ingredients:

4 pieces Egg

100 ml (3 ½ fl. oz.) Almond milk

2 tablespoons Arrowroot powder

4 tablespoons Chestnut flour

1 tablespoon Olive oil (mild)

2 tablespoons Maple syrup

2 tablespoons Cocoa powder

1 tablespoon Coconut oil

1 piece Banana

2 pieces Kiwi (green)

2 pieces Mandarins

Directions:

Mix all ingredients (except fruit and coconut oil) into an even dough.

Melt some coconut oil in a small pan and pour a quarter of the batter into it.

Bake it like a pancake baked on both sides.

Place the fruit in a wrap and serve it lukewarm.

A wonderfully sweet start to the day!

Nutrition:

Calories: 555 kcal

Protein: 20.09 g

Fat: 34.24 g

Carbohydrates: 45.62 g

43 Chocolate Sauce

Preparation Time: 10 minutes

Cooking Time: 10 minutes

Servings: 2 cups

Ingredients:

75 g Cocoa powder

250 ml Coconut milk (can)

95 pieces Dates

3 tablespoon Coconut oil

½ teaspoon Vanilla extract

1 pinch Salt

Directions:

Put the dates in a bowl, pour boiling water over them and let them stand for 10 minutes.

Drain the dates.

Heat the coconut milk and coconut oil in a pan.

Place all the ingredients in a blender and puree into an even sauce.

Add some hot water if you think the sauce is too thick. (Mix them again if you add water).

Nutrition:

Calories: 254 Cal

Fat: 45.68 g

Carbs: 56 g

Protein: 28.15 g

Fiber: 59.6 g

44   Hot Sauce

Preparation Time: 10 minutes

Cooking Time: 15 minutes

Servings: 1 cup

Ingredients: 2 pieces Tomato

2 pieces Red peppers

10 cloves Garlic

2 pieces Red pepper

250 ml White wine vinegar

2 tablespoons Olive oil

1 tablespoon Honey

1 tablespoon Celtic sea salt

Directions:

Singe the tomatoes and peppers over your gas burner. (or in the oven at 220 ° C if you don't have a gas burner)

Let cool down.

Cut the paprika into pieces and remove the stones.

Heat a pan and roast the garlic (without oil) for a few minutes. Let cool down.

Clean the peppers, remove the seeds if necessary.

Put the tomatoes, peppers, garlic and peppers in a blender.

Add 125 ml of water and puree well.

Pour the mixture into a saucepan and add the oil, honey, salt, and vinegar. Bring the mixture to a boil. Turn the heat down as soon as it boils and let it simmer for 5 minutes.

Let cool and check if the sauce still needs salt.

Put the sauce in a glass and let it rest in the fridge for 2 days. Thereupon she will soon burst with taste.

Before use; take a bowl and put a fine sieve on it. Pour the sauce over the sieve and press as far as possible with the convex side of the spoon.

You can throw away the residues remaining in the sieve.

Nutrition:

Calories: 338 Cal

Fat: 28.06 g

Carbs: 45.31 g

Protein: 5.9 g

Fiber: 3.9 g

45 Paleo Breakfast Salad With Egg

Preparation Time: 10 minutes

Cooking Time: 5 minutes

Servings: 2 - 3

Ingredients:

1 teaspoon Ghee

2 pieces Egg

1 hand Spinach

½ pieces Red bell pepper

¼ pieces Onion

50 g Carrot

50 g Cucumber

1 piece Tomato

½ pieces Avocado

Directions:

Slice the onion, cut the bell pepper into strips, cut the cucumber and avocado into cubes, grate the carrot and cut the tomato into wedges.

Melt the ghee in a pan over medium heat and beat the eggs into the pan.

In the meantime, prepare the salad by putting all the

remaining ingredients on a plate.

Remove the eggs from the pan when the egg yolk is still a little soft, this looks like a delicious dressing! (or if you prefer a well-fried egg, drizzle your salad with some olive oil as a dressing).

Season with salt and pepper.

Nutrition:

Calories: 236 Cal

Fat: 49.36 g

Carbs: 55.41 g

Protein: 26.54 g

Fiber: 19.1 g

46   Caesar Dressing

Preparation Time: 10 minutes

Cooking Time: 5 minutes

Servings: 1 cup

Ingredients:

250 ml Olive oil

2 tablespoons Lemon juice

4 pieces Anchovy fillet

2 tablespoon Mustard yellow

1 clove Garlic

1/2 teaspoon Salt

½ teaspoon Black pepper

Directions:

Remove the peel from the garlic and chop it finely.

Put all ingredients in a blender and puree evenly.

This dressing can be kept in the fridge for about 3 days.

Nutrition:

Calories: 71 Cal

Fat: 2.78 g Carbs: 6.76 g

Protein: 6.38 g Fiber: 2.1 g

47   Basil Dressing

Preparation Time: 10 minutes

Cooking Time: 5 minutes

Servings: 1 cup

Ingredients:

100 g fresh basil

1 pc Shallots

1 clove Garlic

125 ml Olive oil (mild)

2 tbsp White wine vinegar

Directions:

Finely chop the shallot and garlic.

Put the shallot, garlic, basil, olive oil and vinegar in a blender.

Mix it into an even mix.

Season the dressing and season with salt and pepper.

Place the dressing in a clean glass and store in the refrigerator. It stays fresh and tasty for at least 3 days.

Nutrition:

Calories: 33 Cal

Fat: 0.66 g

Carbs: 3.72 g

Protein: 3.35 g

Fiber: 1.7 g

48 Strawberry Sauce

Preparation Time: 15 minutes

Cooking Time: 15 minutes

Servings: 1 cup

Ingredients:

225 g Strawberries

3 tablespoons Coconut blossom sugar

4 tablespoons Honey

125 ml Water

2 teaspoon Arrowroot powder

Directions:

Roughly chop strawberries.

Put the strawberries in a pan with coconut blossom sugar and honey. Place the pan on medium heat.

In the meantime, mix the arrow roots with a whisk in the water. Add this mixture to the strawberries.

Heat the strawberries until they start to bubble and start to thicken. (Not cook!)

Your strawberry sauce is ready after about 15 minutes. Store the sauce in the fridge in a clean glass.

Nutrition:

Calories: 238 Cal Fat: 3.91 g

Carbs: 105.68 g

Protein: 2.81 g Fiber: 5.4 g

49 Fresh Chicory Salad

Preparation Time: 15 minutes

Cooking Time: 5 minutes

Servings: 2 - 3

Ingredients:

1 piece Orange

1 piece Tomato

1/4 pieces Cucumber

1/4 pieces Red onion

Directions:

Cut off the hard stem of the chicory and remove the leaves.

Peel the orange and cut the pulp into wedges.

Cut the tomatoes and cucumbers into small pieces.

Cut the red onion into thin half rings.

Place the chicory boats on a plate, spread the orange wedges, tomato, cucumber and red onion over the boats.

Sprinkle some olive oil and fresh lemon juice on the dish.

Nutrition:

Calories: 73 Cal

Fat: 0.49 g

Carbs: 15.73 g

Protein: 2.68 g

Fiber: 3.5 g

50 Grilled Vegetables And Tomatoes

Preparation Time: 10 minutes

Cooking Time: 10 minutes

Servings: 2 - 3

Ingredients:

1 piece Zucchini

1 piece Eggplant

3 pieces Tomatoes

1 piece Cucumber

Dressing:

4 tablespoons Olive oil

110 ml Orange juice (fresh)

1 tablespoon Apple cider vinegar

1 hand fresh basil

Directions:

Cut all of the vegetables into equally thick slices (about half a centimeter).

Heat the grill pan and fry the zucchini and eggplant.

Season with salt and pepper while the zucchini and eggplant are fried.

Remove the basil leaves from the branches.

Spread the vegetables alternately on a plate.

Add a leaf of basil every now and then.

Mix the ingredients for the dressing and serve the dressing separately on the side.

Nutrition:

Calories: 168 Cal

Fat: 55.53 g

Carbs: 40.39 g

Protein: 7.7 g

Fiber: 18.7 g

51   Steak Salad

Preparation Time: 10 minutes

Cooking Time: 10 minutes

Servings: 2 - 3

Ingredients:

2 pieces Beef steak

2 cloves Garlic

1 piece Red onion

2 pieces Egg

1 hand Cherry tomatoes

2 hands Lettuce

1 piece Avocado

1/2 pieces Cucumber

1 pinch Season white Salt

1 pinch Black pepper

Directions:

Place the steaks in a flat bowl.

Pour the olive oil over the steaks and press the garlic over it. Turn the steaks a few times so that they are covered with oil and garlic.

Cover the meat and let it marinate for at least 1 hour.

Boil eggs.

Heat a grill pan and fry the steaks medium.

Take the steaks out of the pan, wrap them in aluminum foil and let them rest for 5 to 10 minutes.

Spread the lettuce on the plates.

Cut the steaks into slices and place them in the middle of the salad.

Cut the eggs into wedges, the cucumber into half-moons, the red onion into thin half-rings, the cherry tomatoes into halves and the avocado into slices.

Spread this around the steaks.

Sprinkle over the olive oil and white wine vinegar and season with a little salt and pepper.

Nutrition:

Calories: 131 Cal

Fat: 74.9 g

Carbs: 37.09 g

Protein: 23 g

Fiber: 17 g

52 Zucchini Salad With Lemon Chicken

Preparation Time: 1 hour 10 minutes

Cooking Time: 25 minutes

Servings: 2 - 3

Ingredients:

1 piece Zucchini

1 piece yellow zucchini

1 hand Cherry tomatoes

2 pieces Chicken breast

1 piece Lemon

2 tablespoons Olive oil

Directions:

Utilize a meat mallet or a heavy pan to make the chicken fillets as thin as possible.

Put the fillets in a bowl.

Squeeze the lemon over the chicken and add the olive oil. Cover it and let it marinate for at least 1 hour.

Heat a pan over medium-high heat and fry the chicken until cooked through and browned.

Season with salt and pepper.

Make zucchini from the zucchini and put in a bowl.

Quarter the tomatoes and stir in the zucchini.

Slice the chicken fillets diagonally and place them on the salad.

Drizzle the salad with a little olive oil and season with salt and pepper.

Nutrition:

Calories: 125 Cal

Fat: 80.83 g

Carbs: 4.97 g

Protein: 121.48 g

Fiber: 0.4 g

53   Fresh Salad With Orange Dressing

Preparation Time: 10 minutes

Cooking Time: 5 minutes

Servings: 2 - 3

Ingredients:

1 / 2 fruit Salad

1 piece yellow bell pepper

1 piece Red pepper

100 g Carrot (grated)

1 hand Almonds

Dressing:

4 tablespoon Olive oil

110 ml Orange juice (fresh)

1 tablespoon Apple cider vinegar

Directions:

Clean the peppers and cut them into long thin strips.

Tear off the lettuce leaves and cut them into smaller pieces.

Mix the salad with the peppers and the carrots processed with the Julienne peeler in a bowl.

Roughly chop the almonds and sprinkle over the salad.

Mix all the ingredients for the dressing in a bowl. Pour the dressing over the salad just before serving.

Nutrition:

Calories: 158 Cal

Fat: 55.07 g Carbs: 16.84 g

Protein: 2.76 g Fiber: 4.5 g

54 Tomato And Avocado Salad

Preparation Time: 10 minutes

Cooking Time: 5 minutes

Servings: 2 - 3

Ingredients:

1 piece Tomato

1 hand Cherry tomatoes

1/2 pieces Red onion

1 piece Avocado

Taste fresh oregano

1 1 / 2 EL Olive oil

1 teaspoon White wine vinegar

1 pinch Celtic sea salt

Directions:

Cut the tomato into thick slices.

Cut half of the cherry tomatoes into slices and the other half in half.

Cut the red onion into super thin half rings. (or use a mandolin for this)

Cut the avocado into 6 parts.

Spread the tomatoes on a plate, place the avocado on top and sprinkle the red onion over them.

Sprinkle fresh oregano on the salad as desired.

Drizzle olive oil and vinegar on the salad with a pinch of salt.

Nutrition:

Calories: 138 Cal

Fat: 29.65 g

Carbs: 29.86 g

Protein: 5.6 g

Fiber: 15.8 g

55 Arugula With Fruits And Nuts

Preparation Time: 10 minutes

Cooking Time: 5 minutes

Servings: 2 – 3

Ingredients:

75 g Arugula

2 pieces Peach

1/2 pieces Red onion

1 hand Blueberries

Pecans 1 hand

Dressing:

1/2 pieces Peach

65 ml Olive oil

2 tablespoon White wine vinegar

1 sprig fresh basil

1 pinch Salt

1 pinch Black pepper

Directions:

Halve the 2 peaches and remove the core.

Cut the pulp into pieces.

Heat a grill pan and grill the peaches briefly on both sides.

Cut the red onion into thin half rings.

Roughly chop the pecans.

Heat a pan and roast the pecans in it until they are fragrant.

Place the arugula on a plate and spread it over the peaches, red onions, blueberries and roasted pecans.

Place all the ingredients for the dressing in a blender or food processor and mix to an even dressing.

Drizzle the dressing over the salad.

Nutrition:

Calories: 68 Cal

Fat: 0.61 g

Carbs: 13.09 g

Protein: 3.16 g

Fiber: 3.1 g

56   Spinach Salad With Green Asparagus And Salmon

Preparation Time: 10 minutes

Cooking Time: 5 minutes

Servings: 2 - 3

Ingredients:

2 hands Spinach

2 pieces Egg

120 g smoked salmon

100 g Asparagus tips

150 g Cherry tomatoes

Lemon 1/2 pieces

1 teaspoon Olive oil

Directions:

Make the eggs the way you like them.

Heat a pan with a little oil and fry the asparagus tips al dente.

Halve cherry tomatoes.

Place the spinach on a plate and spread the asparagus tips, cherry tomatoes and smoked salmon on top.

Scare, peel and halve the eggs. Add them to the salad.

Squeeze the lemon over the lettuce and drizzle some olive oil over it.

Season the salad with a little salt and pepper.

Nutrition:

Calories: 208 Cal

Fat: 32.92 g Carbs: 33.24 g

Protein: 46.65 g

Fiber: 5.4 g

57   Brunoise Salad

Preparation Time: 10 minutes

Cooking   Time: 5 minutes

Servings: 1

Ingredients:

1 piece Meat tomato

1/2 pieces Zucchini

1/2 pieces Red bell pepper

1 / 2 pieces yellow bell pepper

1/2 pieces Red onion

3 sprigs fresh parsley

1/4 pieces Lemon

2 tablespoons Olive oil

Directions:

Finely dice the tomatoes, zucchini, peppers and red onions to get a brunoise.

Mix all the cubes in a bowl.

Chop parsley and mix in the salad.

Squeeze the lemon over the salad and add the olive oil.

Season with salt and pepper.

Nutrition:

Calories: 268 Cal

Fat: 28.06 g

Carbs: 28.39 g

Protein: 5.64 g

Fiber: 5.4 g

58   Broccoli Salad

Preparation Time: 10 minutes

Cooking Time: 5 minutes

Servings: 1

Ingredients:

1 piece Broccoli

1/2 pieces Red onion

100 g Carrot (grated)

1 hand Red grapes

Dressing:

2 1/2 tablespoon Coconut yogurt

1 tablespoon Water

1 teaspoon Mustard yellow

1 pinch Salt

Directions:

Slice the broccoli into small florets and cook al dente for 5 minutes.

Cut the red onion into thin half rings.

Halve the grapes.

Mix coconut yogurt, water and mustard with a pinch of salt to make an even dressing.

Drain the broccoli and rinse with ice-cold water to stop the cooking process.

Mix the broccoli with the carrot, onion and red grapes in a bowl.

Serve the dressing separately on the side.

Nutrition:

Calories: 91 Cal

Fat: 0.52 g

Carbs: 20.79 g

Protein: 2.41 g

Fiber: 5.4 g

59   Ganache Squares:

Preparation Time: 25 minutes

Cooking Time: 15 minutes plus 2 hours chilling time

Servings: 10

Ingredients:

250 ml Coconut milk (can)

1 1/2 tablespoon Coconut oil

100 g Honey

1/2 teaspoon Vanilla extract

350 g Pure chocolate (> 70% cocoa)

1 pinch Salt

2 hands Pecans

Directions:

Put the coconut milk in a saucepan and heat for 5 minutes over medium heat.

Add the vanilla extract, coconut oil and honey and cook for 15 minutes. Add a pinch of salt and stir well.

Break the chocolate into a bowl and pour the hot coconut milk over it. Continuously stir until all of the chocolate has dissolved in the coconut milk.

In the meantime, roughly chop the pecans. Heat a pan without oil and roast the pecans.

Stir the pecans through the ganache.

Let the ganache cool to room temperature. (You may be able to speed this up by placing the bowl in a bowl of cold water.)

Line a baking tin with a sheet of parchment paper. Pour the cooled ganache into it.

Place the ganache in the refrigerator for 2 hours to allow it to harden.

When the ganache has hardened, you can take it out of the mold and cut it into the desired shape.

Nutrition:

Calories: 141 Cal

Fat: 17.56 g

Carbs: 31 g

Protein: 7.65 g

Fiber: 9.3 g

60   Date Candy

Preparation Time: 25 minutes

Cooking Time: 10 minutes plus chilling time

Servings: 10

Ingredients:

10 pieces Medjoul dates

1 hand Almonds

100 g Pure chocolate (> 70% cocoa)

2 1 / 2 tablespoon Grated coconut

Directions:

Melt chocolate in a water bath.

Roughly chop the almonds.

In the meantime, cut the dates lengthways and take out the core.

Fill the resulting cavity with the roughly chopped almonds and close the dates again.

Place the dates on a sheet of parchment paper and pour the melted chocolate over each date.

Sprinkle the grated coconut over the chocolate dates.

Place the dates in the fridge so the chocolate can harden.

Nutrition:

Calories: 292 Cal

Fat: 2.07 g

Carbs: 39 g

Protein: 4.31 g

Fiber: 8.8 g

61   Paleo Bars With Dates And Nuts

Preparation Time: 25 minutes

Cooking Time: 15 minutes

Servings: 15

Ingredients:

180 g Dates

60 g Almonds

60 g Walnuts

50 g Grated coconut

1 teaspoon Cinnamon

Directions:

Roughly cut the dates and soak them in warm water for 15 minutes.

In the meantime, roughly chop the almonds and walnuts.

Drain the dates.

Place the dates with the nuts, coconut and cinnamon in the food processor and mix to an even mass. (but not too long, crispy pieces or nuts make it particularly tasty)

Roll out the mass on 2 baking trays to form an approx. 1 cm thick rectangle.

Cut the rectangle into bars and keep each bar in a piece of parchment paper.

Nutrition:

Calories: 126 Cal

Fat: 69.92 g

Carbs: 160 g

Protein: 26.7 g

Fiber: 27.9 g

62 Banana Strawberry Milkshake

Preparation Time: 15 minutes

Cooking Time: 5 minutes plus chilling time

Servings: 2

Ingredients:

2 pieces Banana (frozen)

1 hand Strawberries (frozen)

250 ml Coconut milk (can)

Directions:

Skin the bananas, slice them and place them in a bag or on a tray. Put them in the freezer the night before.

Put all ingredients in the blender and mix to an even milkshake.

Spread on the glasses.

Nutrition:

Calories: 4 Cal

Fat: 0.04 g

Carbs: 0.92 g

Protein: 0.08 g

Fiber: 0.2 g

63 Buns With Chicken And Cucumber

Preparation Time: 25 minutes

Cooking Time: 20 minutes

Servings: 12

Ingredients:

12 slices Chicken Breast (Spread)

1 piece Cucumber

1 piece Red pepper

50 g fresh basil

3 tablespoons Olive oil

3 tablespoons Pine nuts

Garlic 1 clove

Directions:

Wash the cucumber and cut into thin strips, then cut the peppers into thin strips.

Put the basil, olive oil, pine nuts and garlic in a food processor. Stir to an even pesto.

Season the pesto and season with salt and pepper if necessary.

Place a slice of chicken fillet on a plate, brush with 1 teaspoon of pesto and top the strips with cucumber and peppers.

Carefully roll up the chicken fillet to create a nice roll.

If necessary, secure the rolls with a cocktail skewer.

Nutrition:

Calories: 240 Cal

Fat: 36 g Carbs: 10.69 g

Protein: 72 g

Fiber: 3 g

64   Hazelnut Balls

Preparation Time: 15 minutes

Cooking Time: 10 minutes plus chilling time

Servings: 15 balls

Ingredients:

130 g Dates

140 g Hazelnuts

2 tablespoon Cocoa powder

1/2 teaspoon Vanilla extract

1 teaspoon Honey

Directions:

Place the hazelnuts in a food processor and grind them until you get hazelnut flour (of course you can also use ready-made hazelnut flour).

Put the hazelnut flour in a bowl and set aside.

Put the dates in the food processor and grind them until you get a ball.

Add the hazelnut flour, vanilla extract, cocoa and honey and pulse until you get a nice and even mix.

5

Remove the mixture from the food processor and turn it into beautiful balls.

Store the balls in the fridge.

Nutrition:

Calories: 130 Cal

Fat: 86.97 g

Carbs: 133 g

Protein: 26.09 g

Fiber: 27.2 g

65 Stuffed Eggplants

Preparation Time: 20 minutes

Cooking Time: 35 minutes

Servings: 4

Ingredients:

4 pieces Eggplant

3 tablespoons Coconut oil

1 piece Onion

250 g Ground beef

2 cloves Garlic

3 pieces Tomatoes

1 tablespoon Tomato paste

1 hand Capers

1 hand fresh basil

Directions:

Finely chop the onion and garlic. Cut the tomatoes into cubes and shred the basil leaves.

Bring a large pot of water to a boil, add the eggplants and let it cook for about 5 minutes.

Drain, let cool slightly and remove the pulp with a spoon (leave a rim about 1 cm thick around the skin). Cut the pulp finely and set aside.

Put the eggplants in a baking dish.

Preheat the oven to 175 ° C.

Heat 3 tablespoons of coconut oil in a pan on a low flame and glaze the onion.

Add the minced meat and garlic and fry until the beef is loose.

Add the finely chopped eggplants, tomato pieces, capers, basil and tomato paste and fry them on the pan with the lid for 10 minutes.

Season with salt and pepper.

Fill the eggplant with the beef mixture and bake in the oven for about 20 minutes.

Nutrition:

Calories: 151 Cal

Fat: 72.89 g

Carbs: 147.52 g

Protein: 91.16 g

Fiber: 69.2 g

66 Chicken Teriyaki With Cauliflower Rice

Preparation Time: 45 minutes

Cooking Time: 4 hours

Servings: 8

Ingredients:

500 g Chicken breast

90 ml Coconut amino

2 tablespoons Coconut blossom sugar

1 tablespoon Olive oil

1 teaspoon Sesame oil

50 g fresh ginger

2 cloves Garlic

250 g Chinese cabbage

1 piece Leek

2 pieces Red peppers

1 piece Cauliflower (rice)

1 piece Onion

1 teaspoon Ghee

50 g fresh coriander

1 piece Lime

Directions:

Cut the chicken into cubes. Mix coconut amino, coconut blossom sugar, olive oil and sesame oil in a small bowl.

Finely chop the ginger and garlic and add to the marinade. Put the chicken in the marinade in the fridge overnight.

Roughly cut Chinese cabbage, leek, garlic and paprika and add to the slow cooker. Finally add the marinated chicken and let it cook for about 2 to 4 hours.

When the chicken is almost ready, you can cut the cauliflower into small florets. Then put the florets in a food processor and pulse briefly to prepare rice.

Finely chop an onion, heat a pan with a teaspoon of ghee

and fry the onion. Then add the cauliflower rice and fry briefly.

Spread the chicken and cauliflower rice on the plates and garnish with a little chopped coriander and a wedge of lime.

Nutrition:

Calories: 280 Cal

Fat: 105 g

Carbs: 75 g

Protein: 25 g

Fiber: 21 g

67   Curry Chicken With Pumpkin Spaghetti

Preparation Time: 45 minutes

Cooking Time: 4 hours

Servings: 8

Ingredients:

500 g Chicken breast

2 teaspoons Chili powder

1 piece Onion

1 clove Garlic

2 teaspoons Ghee

3 tablespoon Curry powder

500 ml Coconut milk (can)

200 g Pineapple

200 g Mango

1 piece Red pepper

1 piece Butternut squash

25 g Spring onion

25 g fresh coriander

Directions:

Cut the chicken into strips and season with pepper, salt and chili powder.

Then put the chicken in the slow cooker.

Finely chop the onion and garlic and lightly fry with 2 teaspoons of ghee.

Then add the curry powder.

Deglaze with the coconut milk after a minute.

Add the sauce to the slow cooker along with the pineapple, mango cubes and chopped peppers and let it cook for 2 to 4 hours.

Cut the pumpkin into long pieces and make spaghetti out of it with a spiralizer (that's not easy, it works better with a carrot).

Briefly fry the pumpkin spaghetti in the pan and spread the chicken curry on top.

Garnish with thinly sliced spring onions and chopped coriander.

Nutrition:

Calories: 328 Cal

Fat: 51 g

Carbs: 92 g

Protein: 113 g

Fiber: 20.3 g

68   French Style Chicken Thighs

Preparation Time: 45 minutes

Cooking Time: 4 hours

Servings: 8

Ingredients:

700 g Chicken leg

1 tablespoon Olive oil

2 pieces Onion

4 pieces Carrot

2 cloves Garlic

8 stems Celery

25 g fresh rosemary

25 g Fresh thyme

25 g fresh parsley

Directions:

Season the chicken with olive oil, pepper and salt and rub it into the meat.

Roughly cut onions, carrots, garlic and celery and add to the slow cooker.

Place the chicken on top and finally sprinkle a few sprigs of rosemary, thyme and parsley on top. Let it cook for at least four

hours.

Serve with a delicious salad, enjoy your meal!

Nutrition:

Calories: 122 Cal

Fat: 45.96 g

Carbs: 58.78 g

Protein: 142 g

Fiber: 18.5 g

69 Spicy Ribs With Grilled Vegetables

Preparation Time: 20 minutes

Cooking Time: 20 minutes

Servings: 5

Ingredients:

400 g Spare ribs

4 tablespoons Coconut-Aminos

2 tablespoons Honey

1 tablespoon Olive oil

50 g Spring onions

Garlic 2 cloves

1 piece green chili peppers

1 piece Onion

1 piece Red pepper

1 piece Red pepper

For the roasted pumpkin:

Pumpkin 1 piece

Coconut oil 1 tablespoon

Paprika powder 1 tsp

Directions:

Marinate the ribs the day before. Cut the ribs into pieces with four ribs each. Place the coconut amino, honey and olive oil in a mixing bowl and mix. Chop the spring onions, garlic and green peppers and add them. Spread the ribs on plastic containers and pour the marinade over them. Leave them in the fridge overnight. Cut the onions, peppers and peppers into pieces and put them in the slow cooker. Spread the ribs, including the marinade, and let them cook for at least 4 hours.

Preheat the oven to 200 ° C for the pumpkin.

Cut the pumpkin into moons and place on a baking sheet lined with parchment paper.

Spread a tablespoon of coconut oil on the baking sheet and season with paprika, pepper and salt. Roast the pumpkin in the oven for about 20 minutes and serve with the spare ribs.

Nutrition:

Calories: 151 Cal

Fat: 105 g Carbs: 68.85 g

Protein: 80.34 g Fiber: 6 g

70 Roast Beef With Grilled Vegetables

Preparation Time: 30 minutes

Cooking Time: 50 minutes

Servings: 8

Ingredients:

500 g Roast beef

1 clove Garlic (pressed)

1 teaspoon fresh rosemary

400 g Broccoli

200 g Carrot

400 g Zucchini

4 tablespoons Olive oil

Directions:

Rub the roast beef with freshly ground pepper, salt, garlic and rosemary.

Heat a grill pan over high heat and grill the roast beef for about 20 minutes or until the meat shows nice brown marks on all sides.

Then wrap in aluminum foil and let it rest for a while.

Cut the roast beef into thin slices before serving.

Preheat the oven to 205 ° C. Put all the vegetables in a baking dish.

Drizzle the vegetables with a little olive oil and season with curry powder and / or chili flakes. Put in the oven and bake for 30 minutes or until the vegetables are done.

Nutrition:

Calories: 165 Cal

Fat: 35 g

Carbs: 44.14 g

Protein: 158.84 g

Fiber: 21 g

71 Vegan Thai Green Curry

Preparation Time: 45 minutes

Cooking Time: 4 hours

Servings: 8

Ingredients:

2 pieces green chilies

1 piece Onion

1 clove Garlic

1 teaspoon fresh ginger (grated)

25 g fresh coriander

1 teaspoon Ground caraway

1 piece Lime (juice)

1 teaspoon Coconut oil

500 ml Coconut milk

1 piece Zucchini

1 piece Broccoli

1 piece Red pepper

For the cauliflower rice:

1 teaspoon Coconut oil

1 piece Cauliflower

Directions:

For cauliflower rice, cut the cauliflower into florets and place in the food processor. Pulse briefly until rice has formed. Put aside.

Cut the green peppers, onions, garlic, fresh ginger and coriander into large pieces and combine with the caraway seeds and the juice of 1 lime in a food processor or blender and mix to an even paste.

Heat a pan over medium heat with a teaspoon of coconut oil and gently fry the pasta. Deglaze with coconut milk and add to the slow cooker.

Cut the zucchini into pieces, the broccoli in florets, the peppers into cubes and put in the slow cooker. Simmer for 4 hours. Briefly heat the cauliflower rice in 1 teaspoon of coconut oil, season with a little salt and pepper in a pan over medium heat.

Nutrition:

Calories: 198 Cal

Fat: 10.15 g Carbs: 26.92 g

Protein: 5.76 g Fiber: 6.6 g

72   Indian Yellow Curry

Preparation Time: 45 minutes

Cooking Time: 4 hours

Servings: 8

Ingredients:

2 pieces Onion

1 clove Garlic

300 g Chicken breast

2 teaspoon Coconut oil

1 tablespoon Curry powder

1 teaspoon fresh ginger

1 teaspoon dried turmeric

Laos 1 tsp

500 ml Coconut milk

For the salad:

250 g Iceberg lettuce

1/2 pieces Cucumber

2 pieces Red peppers

25 g Dried coriander

Directions:

Heat a saucepan over medium heat and let the coconut oil melt. Finely chop onions and clove of garlic. Put in the pot and add the herbs, deglaze with the coconut milk and stir well.

Cut the chicken into cubes and add to the slow cooker along with the curry sauce and let it cook for 4 hours.

Cut iceberg lettuce, spread cucumber and bell pepper cubes over it and season with the coriander. Serve the salad with the curry.

Nutrition:

Calories: 118 Cal

Fat: 39.18 g Carbs: 48.04 g

Protein: 72.04 g

Fiber: 14.3 g

73   Sweet Potato Hash Browns

Preparation Time: 20 minutes

Cooking Time: 15 minutes

Servings: 8

Ingredients:

1 pinch Celtic sea salt

1 tablespoon Coconut oil

2 pieces Sweet potato

2 pieces Red onion

2 teaspoons Balsamic vinegar

1 piece Apple

125 g lean bacon strips

Directions:

Clean the red onions and cut them into half rings.

Heat a pan with a little coconut oil over medium heat. Fry the onion until it's almost done.

Add the balsamic vinegar and a pinch of salt and cook until the balsamic vinegar has boiled down. Put aside.

Skin the sweet potatoes and cut them into approx. 1.5 cm cubes.

Heat the coconut oil in a pan and fry the sweet potato cubes for 10 minutes.

Add the bacon strips for the last 2 minutes and fry them until you're done.

Cut the apple into cubes and add to the sweet potato cubes.

Let it roast for a few minutes.

Then add the red onion and stir well.

Spread the sweet potato hash browns on 2 plates.

Nutrition:

Calories: 104 Cal

Fat: 58.46 g

Carbs: 122 g Protein: 18.16 g

Fiber: 15.8 g

74 Tuna Salad In Red Chicory

Preparation Time: 10 minutes

Cooking Time: 5 minutes

Servings: 2

Ingredients:

4 pieces Red chicory

160 g Tuna (tin)

1 piece Orange

1 tablespoon fresh parsley (finely chopped.)

5 pieces Radish

1 / 2 TL Apple cider vinegar

Directions:

Drain the tuna.

Cut the orange into wedges and cut them into small pieces.

Cut radishes into small pieces.

Mix all the ingredients (except the red chicory) in a small bowl. Season with salt and pepper

Spread the tuna salad on the red chicory leaves.

Nutrition:

Calories: 243 Cal

Fat: 3.26 g

Carbs: 69.53 g

Protein: 41.36 g

Fiber: 27.2 g

75 Paleolicious Smoothie Bowl

Preparation Time: 10 minutes

Cooking Time: 5 minutes

Servings: 1

Ingredients:

1 piece Banana (frozen)

1 hand Spinach

1/2 pieces Mango

1/2 pieces Avocado

100 ml Almond milk

For garnish:

Mango1/2 pieces

Raspberries1 hand

Grated coconut1 tablespoon

Walnuts (roughly chopped) 1 tablespoon

Directions:

Mix all ingredients in a blender and mix to an even mass.

Put the mixture in a bowl and garnish with the remaining ingredients.

Of course, you can vary the garnish as you wish.

Nutrition:

Calories: 157 Cal

Fat: 35.38 g

Carbs: 67.88 g

Protein: 8.71 g

Fiber: 19.4 g

76 Granola

Preparation Time: 30 min

Cooking Time: 0 min

Servings: 1

Ingredients:

1 cup buckwheat puffs

1 cup buckwheat flakes (ready to eat type, but not whole buckwheat that needs to be cooked) ½ cup coconut flakes

½ cup Medjool dates, without pits, chopped into smaller, bite-sized pieces

1 cup of cacao nibs or very dark chocolate chips

1/2 cup walnuts, chopped

1 cup strawberries, chopped and without stems 1 cup plain Greek, or coconut or soy yogurt.

Directions:

Mix, without yogurt and strawberry toppings. You can store for up to a week. Store in an airtight container. Add toppings (even different berries or different yogurt. You can even use the berry toppings as you will learn how to make from other recipes.

Nutrition: Calories: 69 Cal

Fat: 29.39 g Carbs: 103.04 g

Protein: 18.67 g

Fiber: 15.4 g

77 Yogurt With Dark Chocolate, Chopped Walnuts, And Mixed Berries/Coconut Or Soy Yogurt With Chopped Walnuts, Mixed Berries, And Dark Chocolate

Preparation Time: 5 minutes

Cooking Time: 5 minutes

Servings: 1

Ingredients:

about 11/3 cups (125g) mixed berries

2/3 cup (150g) plain Greek yogurt (or vegan alternative, such as soy or coconut yogurt)

1/4 cup (25g) walnuts, chopped

11/2 tablespoons (10g) dark chocolate (85 percent cocoa solids), grated

Directions:

Simply add your preferred berries to a bowl and top with the yogurt.

Sprinkle with the walnuts and chocolate.

Nutrition:

Calories: 196 Cal

Fat: 59.23 g

Carbs: 345 g

Protein: 25.19 g

Fiber: 15.7 g

78 Buckwheat Pancakes With Dark Chocolate, Strawberries And Crushed Walnuts

Preparation Time: 15 minutes

Cooking Time: 15 minutes

Servings: 6 - 8

Ingredients:

For the Chocolate Sauce

1 tbsp. Extra virgin olive oil

3.5 oz (85% cocoa solids) - Dark chocolate

1 tbsp. Double cream

85ml milk

For the Pancakes

1 cup Buckwheat Flour

350ml milk

1 Large Egg

1 tbsp Extra Virgin Olive Oil for Cooking

To Serve

Walnuts - ½ cup (chopped)

Strawberries – 2 cups (hulled and chopped)

Directions:

Get your pancake batter by placing all the ingredients for the pancakes minus the olive oil in a blender. Blend until smooth. Your mixture should not be too runny or too thick. If you have any excess batter, transfer it to an airtight container and keep in the fridge for a maximum of 5 days. Mix thoroughly before you use it.

To get your chocolate sauce, place a heatproof bowl over a pan of simmering water, place the chocolate in the bowl to melt. Add the milk into the bowl once the chocolate is melted, whisk thoroughly, then add the olive oil and double cream. Leave the water in the pan simmering on the lowest heat until your pancake is ready – this will keep the sauce warm.

To make the pancakes, place a heavy-bottomed frypan on medium heat until it begins to smoke, then add the olive oil. Add some of the pancake batters into the center of the pan, then tip the excess batter around the pan until the entire surface is covered. Add a little more batter if needed. Cook the pancake for approx. one minute on each side so long as your pan is hot enough.

Once the pancake begins to go brown around the edges, use a spatula to loosen it around its edges before flipping it over. Gently fry in one direction so that the pancake does not break.

Cook for one more minute on the other side before transferring the pancakes to a plate.

Add some strawberries in the center of the pancake and then roll up the pancake. Repeat this until you have enough pancakes.

Spread enough sauce on the pancakes, then sprinkle over some of the chopped walnuts.

At first, your pancakes may fall apart or come out too fat, but as you continue, you will find the consistency that is best for you.

Nutrition:

Calories: 247 Cal

Fat: 78.48 g

Carbs: 171 g

Protein: 32.92 g

Fiber: 30.3 g

CHAPTER 10:

Maintenance

Food cravings would be the dieter's worst enemy. All these are an extreme or uncontrollable desire for certain foods, even stronger than your regular appetite. The different types of foods that folks crave are tremendously changeable, but all these are processed junk foods that have a lot of sugar.

Cravings are among the primary reasons why people struggle to lose weight and keep it away.

Here are 10 simple techniques to check or prevent unhealthy sugar and food cravings.

1. Drink water

Thirst can be confused with food or hunger cravings. In case you're feeling that sudden urge to get a particular food, try drinking a huge glass of water and then wait for a couple of minutes. You might discover that the craving disappears as your body was actually only thirsty.

2. Eat protein

Eating more protein can lower your appetite and prevent you from overeating. Additionally, it additionally reduces cravings and can help you feel satisfied.

One analysis of obese teenage girls showed that eating a high protein breakfast reduced cravings somewhat. Still another study in obese guys revealed that increasing dietary intake to 25 percent of carbs decreased cravings by 60 percent. In addition, the urge to eat during the night-time has been decreased by 50 percent.

Increasing protein intake can reduce cravings by up to 60 percent and slice off the urge to snack during the night by 50 percent.

3. Distance yourself in the craving

When you're feeling that craving, make an effort to distance yourself from it. For example, you'll be able to have a brisk walk or perhaps a shower to alter the mind onto something different. A big change in environment and thought might help block the craving. Some studies also have demonstrated that nicotine gum might help decrease cravings and appetite. Decrease the urge by chewing-gum, going on a walk or just taking a shower.

4. Plan meals

If possible, attempt to organize your diet daily or weekly. By already understanding what you are going to consume, you get rid of the variable of spontaneity and doubt.

In case that you do not need to consider everything to eat at the subsequent meal, you may soon be less enticed and not as inclined to undergo migraines. Planning your meals eliminates spontaneity and doubt, each that could result in cravings.

5. Avoid getting unbelievably hungry

Hunger is among the primary reasons why people experience cravings. To avoid becoming severely hungry, it could possibly be a very good plan to eat regularly and have healthy snacks close at hand. By being ready, and preventing lengthy periods of appetite, you could have the ability to protect against the cravings. Hunger is a significant cause of cravings. Steer clear of extreme hunger by constantly using a healthful snack ready.

6. Fight stress

Stress may cause cravings for food and influence eating behaviors, mainly for ladies.

Women under stress are demonstrated to eat more calories and also experience greater cravings compared to non-stressed ladies.

Moreover, stress increases your blood levels of cortisol, a hormone that could allow you to gain weight, mainly in the gut area.

Try to minimize stress in your environment by addressing it early, meditating and generally, slowing down. Being under stress can cause cravings, eating and weight increase, particularly in women.

7. Ingest spinach extract

Spinach extract is just a "fresh" nutritional supplement available on the current market created by spinach leaves. It helps postpone fat digestion which raises the degree of hormones that reduce appetite and craving, for example as for instance, studies reveal that taking 3.7--5 g of spinach extract with dinner can decrease cravings and appetite for many hours.

One study in obese girls revealed that the 5 g of spinach extract each day reduced cravings for chocolate and also spicy foods by way a whopping 87—95 percent. Spinach extract aids in the digestion of fat and also increases the degree of hormones which may decrease cravings and appetite.

8. Get enough sleep

Your appetite is mainly affected by the hormones that change during the day. Sleep deprivation disrupts changes and could lead to poor regulation of appetite and strong cravings. Studies support this, revealing that sleep-deprived men and women are up to 55 percent more likely to gain weight, in comparison to folks who have enough sleep.

To explore this rationale, getting a good night's sleep could possibly be one of the most powerful tactics to protect against cravings for unsafe food choices.

Sleep deprivation may interrupt ordinary changes in the hormones of desire, resulting in cravings and poor control of appetite.

9. Eat proper meals

Hunger and also a scarcity of important nutrients may cause cravings that are certain.

Consequently, it is critical to eat healthful foods at mealtimes. In this manner, the entire body receives the nutrients it takes, and you also won't feel exceptionally hungry following ingestion.

In case you also end up needing a snack between meals, make sure it's something healthy. Grab whole foods, like fruits, nuts, seeds or vegetables. Eating proper foods aids in preventing cravings and appetite, while also making certain your entire body receives the nutrients it takes.

10. Exercise mindful eating

Mindful eating is all about practicing mindfulness, a kind of meditation, even in regard to eating and foods. Additionally, it instructs one to produce a comprehension of one's diet plan, feelings, appetite and cravings, and bodily senses.

Mindful eating educates one to distinguish between cravings and also actual hunger. It makes it possible to select your answer, rather than acting on it thoughtlessly or impulsively.

Eating psychotherapy entails being present as you eat, slowing and chewing thoroughly. It's likewise essential to steer clear of distractions, just like the television or your own smartphone.

One 6-week study in binge-eaters unearthed that cautious eating reduced binge eating episodes by four to 1.5 a week. In addition, it decreased the urgency of every occurrence.

CHAPTER 11:

7 Day Meal Plan

DAYS	BREAKFAST	LUNCH	DINNER
PHASE 1			
1	The Sirtfood Green Juice	Chicken Teriyaki With Cauliflower Rice	Yogurt With Dark Chocolate, Chopped Walnuts, And Mixed Berries/Coconut Or Soy Yogurt With Chopped Walnuts, Mixed Berries, And Dark Chocolate
2	Buckwheat Pancakes With Dark Chocolate, Strawberries And Crushed Walnuts	Salmon With Capers And Lemon	Salad With Bacon, Cranberries And Apple
3	Avocado And Salmon Salad Buffet	Roast Beef With Grilled Vegetables	Apple Cinnamon Wraps
PHASE 2			
4	Paleo Breakfast Salad With Egg	Curry Chicken With Pumpkin Spaghetti	Date Candy
5	Granola	Zucchini Salad With Lemon Chicken	Paleo-Force Bars
6	Paleolicious Smoothie Bowl	Brunoise Salad	Stuffed Eggplants
7	Sweet And Sour Pan With Cashew Nuts	Fresh Chicory Salad	Ganache Squares

Having seen those regularly significant alterations ourselves firsthand, we understand the amount you'll have to not merely hold all the one's benefits, anyway, observe stunningly better results. Sirtfoods are intended to be eaten forever. The inquiry is how you adjust what you have been doing in Phase 1 into your common dietary repeating. That is what initiated us to make a subsequent fourteen-day remodel plan intended to assist you with making the change from Phase 1 to your additional ordinary dietary daily practice and therefore help keep up and also increment the benefits of the Sirtfood Diet.

What's in store

During Phase 2, you will merge your weight reduction outcomes and hold them to get in shape consistently.

Recollect that the central striking angle we have found with the Sirtfood Diet is that greatest or the entirety of the weight that individuals lose is from fats, and that numerous genuinely put on a couple of muscle. So we have to remind you again now not to pick your advancement absolutely by methods for the numbers on the scale. Search inside the imitate to find on the off chance that you are looking more slender and extra conditioned, perceive how your garments are fitting, and slurp up the commendations that you may get from others.

Recall too that primarily as the weight reduction will save, the wellness benefits will develop. By following the fourteen-day protection plan, you're entirely beginning to put down the standards for a fate of profoundly rooted wellbeing.

The most effective method to FOLLOW PHASE 2

The way to accomplishment in this stage is to keep up pressing your eating routine loaded with Sirtfoods. To make it as spotless as could reasonably be expected, we've assembled a seven-day menu plan which will follow, including flavorful family-accommodating projects, with consistently pressed to the rafters with Sirtfoods (however observe page 149 for guidance concerning kids). You should simply rehash the seven-day procedure twice to complete the fourteen days of Phase 2.

The end of the first phase of the sirtfood diet marks phase two. This phase is all about the maintenance and regulation of the diet that you have initially started. As the first phase prepares the body to accept the dietary changes and work accordingly, the second phase is the result yielding stage, provided that the dieter follows it in an appropriate manner. This phase allows the body to continue working towards the weight loss goals in a steady and progressive manner. That is the reason that the overall duration of the stage is nearly two weeks.

In this second phase, there is no such caloric restriction as it is in the case of the first phase. In this phase, as long as the dieter is consuming food that is rich in sirtuins for three times a day, it is considered appropriate to achieve all the weight loss goals, because by now the body is already tuned as a result of the first phase. Instead of consuming green juices about three -two times per day, the dieter can now drink one glass of juice a day, and that will be enough to maintain the accelerated rates of metabolism. When to take the juice depends on you, either to take the juice after the meal or before it.

CHAPTER 12:

Shopping Tips

B eing a little more particular regarding the foods that you buy at the store will be able to assist you to get right back on the right track after eating unhealthily isn't difficult. Examine the food labels – the ingredients – so that you are able to make a more informed decision regarding whether it belongs in your eating plan. Chen states it mainly crucial to pay careful attention to serving sizes. "A jar of juice might actually comprise two portions," she states. This means it includes twice the calories and sugar than what's recorded on the label. Also, as you are not likely in the habit of just drinking half a juice, this will prevent you from losing weight. Other critical elements to consider will be the total amount of protein and fiber in meals. Take 2 g of fiber and 20 g of protein into every meal to feel full and satisfied.

The best solution to stop cravings happening at the store will be always to go once you've eaten. Never ever proceed to the supermarket famished. Eating prior to going to the supermarket may help reduce the danger of unwelcome cravings and spontaneous buying.

By far, the best way to load up on those sirtfoods is to start your day with a healthy smoothie. Especially a green one as it's a great refreshing kick start to your body and you can easily pack in 5Fruits/vegetables in one drink. It's sure to keep hunger away too!

We've provided lots of recipes for smoothies which you can not only have for breakfast but as a lunch replacement or mid-day snack. Bear in mind that although the recipes have been categorized as breakfast, light bites and main meals etc. You are free to swap them around.

If you have had a busy day and haven't been able to pack in the sirt goodies as much as you would like, you can always supplement with a handful of walnuts, a green tea or a coffee in between meals to give you a boost and keep hunger away.

If you are careful with your calorie intake, you can be guided by the information on each recipe. A little word of caution when it comes to dates or 'nature's toffees' as some people call them – they are rich in calories. One date contains around 61 calories, so don't go overboard. That said, if you would normally reach for cakes, sweets or biscuits then a date or two is a good substitute because you won't be consuming empty refined sugar calories, yet still enjoying a sweet treat.

If you haven't already, swap your normal cup for green tea which has virtually zero calories. If you don't have a taste for it, you can try it with a flavoring such as jasmine, or even try the recipe for iced cranberry green tea for a refreshing way to drink it. Matcha, which is a type of green tea, is an even stronger tea which also comes in a powder which can be added to smoothies and cooking. Health shops stock matcha, or alternatively, you can buy it online.

Keep a parsley plant on your window ledge because you can add it to virtually anything or even nibble on a sprig! Lovage is a relative of parsley, which has even greater sirtuin-activating benefits, so if you can find it (and it's a big if) use that instead of parsley. Because it's not so easy to find, we have not included lovage in any of these recipes, but if you do get hold of some just add it in.

Capers are available in most supermarkets and sold in jars. They do have a strong salty flavor so you won't need to use too many.

When it comes to chocolate, don't be tempted to buy a sugar-laden milk chocolate bar at the check-out because it won't contain much cocoa. Always aim for good quality dark chocolate with a high cocoa content of around 85% cocoa. Yes, it is more bitter, but your taste buds will soon adapt, and a square of chocolate after a meal is a great treat to round off the day.

The eating regimen originates from the writing of a similar name. The creators – Aidan Goggins and Glen Matten – of the sirtfood diet exhort eating for the most part nourishments rich in sirtuins, a sort of protein in plant nourishments. "The eating plan itself is intended to 'turn on' the sirtuin qualities (especially sirt-1), which are accepted to support digestion, increment fat consuming, battle aggravation, and control craving," says Clark.

Early investigations propose that calorie limitation and resveratrol (a polyphenol found in nourishments like grapes, blueberries, and peanuts), initiate the sirt-1 quality, and these two standards support the sirtfood way to deal with eating.

CHAPTER 13:

Q&A Sirt Diet

What's the reason?

It depends on eating a gathering of nourishments that contain something the creators portray as 'sirtuin activators'. Sirtuins are a class of protein, seven of which (sirt1 to sirt7) have been recognized in people. They seem to have a wide scope of jobs in our body, including potential enemies of maturing and metabolic impacts.

As researchers see increasingly about sirtuins, they're getting keen on the job they may play in assisting with turning on those weight reduction pathways that are normally activated by an absence of nourishment and by taking activity. The hypothesis goes that in the event that you can actuate a portion of the seven sirtuins, you could assist with consuming fat and treat weight with less exertion than it takes to follow some different eating regimens or go through hours on the treadmill.

What would you be able to eat on the eating regimen?

There's a rundown of nourishments containing synthetic intensifies that the creators' state switches on sirtuin and wrench up fat consumption while at the same time bringing down hunger (the last most likely through assisting with accomplishing better glucose control).

Is it compelling for weight reduction?

You ought to get in shape essentially on the grounds that you're eating fewer calories, particularly in stage one. Without a doubt, you may consume fat quicker with this eating routine than with 'any old calorie-confined' plan, and you may feel more full. With respect to the creators' case, this eating regimen is 'clinically demonstrated to lose 7lb in seven days'...

Indeed, it's important that so far the eating regimen has just been tried on 40 sound, exceptionally energetic human guinea pigs in an upmarket rec center in London's Knightsbridge. The analyzers lost a normal of 7lb in seven days while demonstrating increments in bulk and vitality. In any case, at that point, given the calorie limitations of that first week, weight reduction may essentially be because of the extraordinary decrease in calories.

Further examinations are expected to distinguish the long haul sway on waistlines – and general wellbeing – and to see whether sirt calorie counters keep the pounds off any more adequately than they would on different eating regimens. We don't yet have the foggiest idea what, assuming any, sway the expansion of sirt foods to our eating regimen really has on our weight.

What's more, will anybody have the option to stay with the repetitiveness of juices and limit themselves to nourishments on the rundown (and be glad to dump their typical cup for green tea) for all time? With respect to the features that recommend you can appreciate dull chocolate and red wine on this eating regimen – well, truly, it is anything but a green light to expend piles of either!

In the event that you have the funds, the tendency and the stomach for it, I'm very certain it will 'attempt' somewhat for the time being, if simply because it's a successful Directions to confine calories. Furthermore, wine and chocolate aside, the rundown, for the most part, comprises of the very nourishments dietitians and nutritionists suggest for good wellbeing (think products of the soil!).

Regardless of whether it functions admirably enough to make it stand separated from a huge number of weight reduction designs that have trodden this tired way before likewise is not yet clear.

Conclusion

Sirtfood diet program is an idea it is possible to embark on, but perhaps not merely for weight loss but also several due procedures indoors and out human body posture.

The plan asserts that eating particular foods can trigger your "lean receptor" pathway and possess you losing seven pounds in 7 days. Foods such as ginseng, dark chocolate, and milk contain a natural compound called polyphenols, which mimic the results of fasting and exercise. Strawberries, red onions, cinnamon, and garlic will also be powerful Sirtfoods. These foods can activate the sirtuin pathway to help enable weight reduction. The science seems appealing. However, the truth is there is very little research to back up these claims. Plus, the guaranteed speed of weight reduction from the very first week is quite quick and perhaps not in accord with the national institute of health safe fat loss recommendations of a couple of pounds each week.

The diet contains two stages:

For the first three of seven days for Phase 1, you've only been drinking three Sirtfood green juices along with a meal full of Sirtfoods for a total of 1000 calories. On days four to seven, you'll drink two green juices along with two meals for a total of 1,500 calories.

Phase 2, on the other hand, is a 14-day maintenance program, although it is designed to keep your shed weight steady (maybe not maintain your current weight). Each day consists of three balanced Sirtfood dishes plus one green juice.

After those three weeks, you are invited to keep on eating a diet full of Sirtfoods and drinking a green juice each day. You can discover several Sirtfood collection of recipes and online on the Sirtfood site.

The Sirtfood Diet is very well may be natural and inorganic. All things considered, natural produce conveys a more extravagant substance of sirtuin-initiating supplements. Recall that the sirtuin-enacting polyphenols found in plant foods are created in light of natural anxieties, and without the exceptional utilization of pesticides, naturally developed produce should fight that a lot harder to prevent and avoid ecological predators. This is probably going to bring about more significant levels of polyphenols being delivered, making natural produce possibly a more impressive Sirtfood than its nonorganic proportionate. While natural is best, you will even now get extraordinary outcomes from the Sirtfood Diet in the event that you decide on inorganic produce.

Is The Sirtfood Diet The Miracle To Lose Weight?

The name is not new, since in the last 10 years the "Sirtfood" (Sirte food) has been on the lips of many dietitians as a remedy for the cellular rejuvenation of our body. But it has been in the last year and a half when it has become fashionable thanks to the fact that two British nutritionists, Aidan Goggin's and Glen Matten , colleagues from the University of Surrey, saw that in addition to helping the regeneration of our body, this diet also helped to weight loss. But what exactly is the "Sirtfood"?

These are foods that indirectly increase the activity of sit-ins, proteins that regulate various biological processes such as aging, cell death, inflammation and metabolism. Hence, prioritizing its consumption can be an aid when it comes to losing weight. According to the researchers, its effects are similar to those caused by fasting, a process during which the energy reserves of our body activate these enzymes (which they describe as the 'skinny gene'). It is then when our fat reserves stop accumulating lipids and our body stops its habitual growth and the "survival" mode is activated.

The most common foods in this diet and that help in this weight loss process are olive oil, red onions, parsley, strawberries, walnuts, apples, capers, dark chocolate or wine.

What Do Other Nutritionists Think?

Although they have received the favor of many colleagues, there are others who warn about their effectiveness. According to them, these types of fast diets in which weight is lost so quickly are not highly recommended, because they ensure that the "rebound effect" will be much stronger once the feeding rhythm that they request is left. The dietician Emer Delaney warns that "in my experience, the first 3 kilos they promise will be of liquids, but burning fat takes time and I am sure that this diet is not possible. A balanced diet with low fat and high protein foods, as well as vegetables and fruit are necessary. " In fact, many of the foods they recommend are already part of a balanced diet.

Be that as it may, if you are thinking of carrying out a diet, always remember to speak to a doctor or specialist beforehand.

Over the course of this reading, you have seen the best sirtfood recipes you can try at home. By learning how to meal plan you will be able to easily master the Sirt food diet with little day-to-day effort required. You will be able to enjoy delicious meals at a moment's notice without having to struggle after a long day of work.

You can trust that the Sirt diet works, as many people have experienced a profound change from the plan. While you may have heard about Adele's fifty-pound loss, there are many less famous people around the world who have had similar success. Give phases one and two a try, just once, and you are sure to see results. If you can commit to trying it out for just those few weeks, then you can feel confident in either maintaining the plan through including sirtfoods in your regular diet. You might even repeat phases one and two for increased weight loss.

The meal plan I provided you will help you get on your feet. Whether you choose to use the plan exactly how I designed, customize it, or create your own from scratch, you will find that by having a plan and guide to follow eating healthier, losing weight and boosting your health can be easier than ever.

There are over 70 recipes in this collection, all of which can help you along every step of your journey to reach your goal.

Whether you start out following the Sirt diet to the letter or simply experimenting and enjoying the dishes in this collection, you are sure to experience benefits and fall in love with food all over again. What are you waiting for? With just a little effort and time in the kitchen, you can get on your way to success.

Made in the USA
Las Vegas, NV
05 December 2020